MW00638834

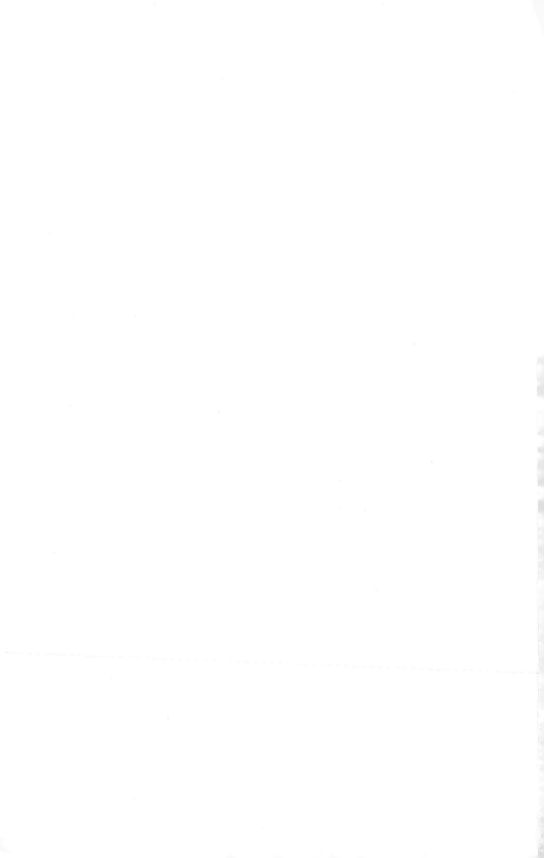

DEEP

BREATHS

A MEMOIR OF A LIFE
FILLED WITH ANXIETY

JOHN LOCKLIN

First published by John Locklin 2023

Copyright © 2023 by John Locklin

All rights reserved. No part of this publication may be reproduced, stored or transmitted in any form or by any means, electronic, mechanical, photocopying, recording, scanning, or otherwise without written permission from the publisher. It is illegal to copy this book, post it to a website, or distribute it by any other means without permission.

John Locklin asserts the moral right to be identified as the author of this work.

John Locklin has no responsibility for the persistence or accuracy of URLs for external or third-party Internet Websites referred to in this publication and does not guarantee that any content on such Websites is, or will remain, accurate or appropriate.

First edition ISBN: 9781088198353

Cover art by Amanda Cestaro

Editing by Caryn Rivadeneira

To all of my family, friends, and unexpected allies,
I thank you now and forever.

Within the pages of this book, I open up about my battles with anxiety and panic attacks. It's important to note that these stories may evoke triggering emotions if you find yourself facing similar challenges.

If, at any point, you feel the need to step back, please know that it's absolutely okay. You can skip a chapter or bookmark your page and set the book aside until you feel ready to dive back in.

Your wellbeing and mental health always come first, and I want you to have a safe and comfortable reading experience.

Please take care of yourself throughout your journey.

U h oh, it's happening...

Nothing even brought this one on...

Hold on tight. Don't let it take control. You've done this a million times.

Just breathe—it will go away. It always does...

...but what if it doesn't?

Am I even breathing? Breathe. Deep Breaths. You are supposed to breathe.

In... 2...3...4...5...

And out ... 2...3...

Oh my god

Oh my god

Oh my godohmygodohmyohmygodohmygodohmygod

Oh my GOD

NO no no no no no no
I have to get **out**
I need to get out of here
I have to **GO**
Run

Run run run

I have to get out of this room. I have to **get out** of here
I have to **get out of my SKIN**

BREATHE.

Breathe....
Just.
Breathe.

Breathing makes me dizzy.

Am I dizzy?
I *am* dizzy.
What if I faint?
What if I **die**?
What if
What if—

No. Just walk.
Walk, walk, walk, just walk

There is nothing to be scared of there is nothing to be scared
of there is nothing to be scared of—

But I can't breathe

I CAN'T BREATHE
Why are my lungs not working?
I don't want to die. I don't want to die. I don't WANT TO DIE.
Shit. Shit shit shit shit shit.

Scream.
You need to SCREAM.

What if this never stops?
What if
What if—

How long have I been holding my breath?

BREATHE.

In and out.
In and out.
In and—

You have to run, you have to run, you—

No.
Breathe.
Breathe...
Breathe..........

It's over.
You did it. It's finally over.

But what if—

"Inhale courage, exhale fear."

- Unknown

Introduction

I hate it when people tell me to "just breathe."

Do they suppose I never thought of that? Well, newsflash, I did. And yes, I *am* actively holding my breath at this very moment, but I am **fully aware** that I'm supposed to breathe.

I have been told by more people and more times than I can count to "just breathe- you will get through it". Saying this is like looking at a crying baby and saying, "Just smile." It doesn't work.

When you have your first panic attack, it's not a matter of forgetting to breathe; it's more like you *can't* breathe. It is like someone put a "Do Not Enter" sign on your airways and your lungs are constricted in a vice. Is it an asthma attack? Nope, sorry. No asthma for you. Wait—do you feel that tingling sensation in your left arm? Your chest tightens, and fear sets in as a wave of nausea washes over you like a rancid seaweed smoothie. You know those symptoms, right? It must be a heart attack.

So, what do you do? You turn to the wise oracle known as Google herself to confirm your suspicions. You type in your symptoms, coaxing the search engine to break the news. And what do you know? It *is* a heart attack, and you're undoubtedly on your deathbed. The world is about to crumble, and the many (or few) years you've spent on this planet are all you'll ever have. You're too young to die, right? At least you can say you lived a good life. Sure, it mainly consisted of binge-watching your favorite shows on Netflix, but that's the norm nowadays.

Although, here's the kicker: you're not dying, and it's not a heart attack. This is a panic attack.

Now, I must admit panic attacks differ from person to person. Some people experience mild episodes as if their anxiety is politely offering a cup of tea rather than barging in like an uninvited relative during the holidays. But for others, panic attacks come in a more extreme package.

Regardless of your panic attack severity, those of us who suffer from them can all agree on one thing:

Panic attacks suck.

Describing a panic attack to someone who hasn't experienced one is like explaining the concept of time to a goldfish. It is an intricate and sloppy dance between heart-pounding horror and mind-numbing fear. It is feeling as if you're on the brink of needing to run from an invisible monster, all while also acknowledging that you don't have anything to be scared of because the monster is not real. Therefore, in theory, you could easily just take a moment to think and rationalize that this big, scary "inevitability" isn't real and can't hurt you. Easy-peasy, right? Panic attacks should be as easy to overcome as blowing your nose to relieve stuffiness.

DEEP BREATHS | 15

They're essentially being scared of nothing, so moving on and banishing them forever should be a piece of cake.

Boy, oh boy, do I wish it were that simple.

I often get asked: "When did your anxiety attacks start?" In truth, I've been dealing with panic attacks for as long as my brain can remember.

According to my mom, they began around four years old.

Growing up, I saw more therapists and psychiatrists than I could count. It was always the same—I was too young for a panic disorder, and medication was reserved for the older and more "experienced" anxiety enjoyers. Instead, I learned about behavioral therapy, coping mechanisms, and, yes, you guessed it, breathing techniques. They're supposed to work like magic—backed by science—and make everything hunky-dory.

Except, my panic attacks didn't exactly get the memo.

Now, at twenty-eight, I've learned a thing or two from my lifelong dance with anxiety. I've discovered that brains are more complicated than I could have ever believed. I've come to understand that fear doesn't require a physical form to be utterly terrifying. And although many people don't grasp the true nature of panic attacks, opening up about my own has revealed that countless others do. Turns out, many, many people share the same mental battles, and contrary to what my brain tries to convince me, I'm never alone in this.

So, the forthcoming pages of this book will be a treasure trove of stories—tales of my lowest lows and moments of triumph. You will hear moments when I swore that even though none of my hundreds of panic attacks so far had killed me, this one would be the exception. But you will also hear moments when the adrenaline subsided, allowing me to look back and think wonder what was going through my mind.

Through reflection, I've come to understand myself better. I've evaluated techniques that work (and those that don't) and, believe it or not, found moments to smile and laugh at the outrageous things my brain conjured up during an attack. Because let's face it: when your mind is a on wild roller coaster ride, sometimes laughter is the best seatbelt you can have.

When the dust settles, and my body stops tingling, the first thing that always comes to mind is, *What the hell was I thinking?* And that is usually followed with a smile. Humor is not just a coping mechanism for me, but in using humor, I have found ways to not be bogged down by my lifelong leech and instead, empower myself by it.

That said, anxiety can also make you feel like the loneliest person in the world, so as we journey through the rest of these pages, I'm here to remind you that you are never alone and that what you're experiencing is entirely normal. You may feel like an outcast or a freak, but let these pages remind you that, without a doubt, there are freakier people than you, even if you get scared at seemingly nothing.

And even if you have never encountered a panic attack yourself, I hope this book and the tips included enlighten you about the realities of an anxiety disorder - going beyond the mere butterflies people get in their stomachs before a nerve-wracking presentation - and provide you with tools to use in the other battles you may face throughout this long journey we call life. Maybe you have seen someone have an attack and felt you had no way to help, or perhaps you have heard of panic attacks and felt they were blown out of proportion. These are logical thoughts. That said, let these stories serve as an eye-opening guide to you.

Regardless of your reasons for reading this book—whether to relate, to feel seen, to understand, or simply because the cover looked fantastic—I'd like to take a moment to remind you:

Just breathe.

"Mental health is not a destination, but a process.
It's about how you drive, not where you're going."

Noam Shpancer

1
What is a Panic Attack?

Panic Attack (noun): an intense attack of anxiety characterized by feelings of impending doom and trembling, sweating, pounding heart, and other physical symptoms.

- Dictionary.com

I hope by now I have thoroughly charmed you with my sparkling personality and irresistible charm, and a little science won't scare you off. In fact, the rest of this chapter is very little science at all, but rather a mix of what I have learned about panic attacks and what is happening in my brain during one. It also attacks the impossible question: "What is a panic attack?"

Panic attacks defy definitions. If you have ever had one, you'll notice that definition up there at the start of this chapter barely cracks the surface of definition. But being equipped with some knowledge of what makes an attack happen makes them a bit more approachable.

Panic attacks are commonly misunderstood or confused with the run-of-the-mill feelings everyone experiences. Everyone gets nervous from time to time, right? In today's day and age it feels like everyone is stressed about something (probably money). It's practically a fact of life.

While these statements hold some truth, panic disorders and panic attacks are much more than that. The pit in your stomach when you think you lost your keys, the butterflies before a presentation, a scary Halloween hay ride through a dark haunted forest? While these feelings can certainly cause panic attacks, often, they don't even hold a candle to a genuine attack.

Some people may have just one panic attack in their entire lives, while others, like yours truly, have lost count. Some folks may even live with generalized anxiety all their lives but never experience a full-blown attack.

And, while everyone feels panic or anxiety from time to time, panic and anxiety *disorders* are entirely different and something that can't just go away.

I may not have an MD after my name, so I'll avoid discussing things beyond my expertise. Instead, I'll shed light on what I've learned about the chemical nuances of panic disorders and panic attacks, how they relate to my life, and my wild ride with anxiety in an attempt to come up with a better definition.

"Just snap out of it."

"There's nothing to be scared of."

"Calm down."

"You're acting like a child."

"You're just seeking attention."

"Change your mindset, and you'll be cured."

I've heard it all. And for the longest time, these words stung because, deep down, I believed them. Why couldn't I make it all stop? There was nothing to fear, so why couldn't I just calm down? My teeth chattered, my arms flailed about, and I couldn't stop screaming—what *was* I? Was I *really* nothing more than a toddler throwing a tantrum? Did I crave attention? How on earth could I just **stop**?

The short answer is: I couldn't be cured or snap out of it because, thanks to a chemical imbalance in my brain, anxiety is something I'll be facing head-on for the rest of my days.

As of today, my official anxiety-related laundry list of a diagnosis reads: Chronic and Severe Panic and Generalized Anxiety Disorder, with panic attacks and a dash of Somatic Symptoms Disorder thrown in for good measure.

You will hear more about the intricacies of my laundry list of diagnoses as we progress through this book. Essentially, though, my diagnosis means that while I can manage my anxiety, there is no magical cure.

Now, I know what you think as you read this: *Great, I'm doomed. These panic attacks are here to stay forever.*

But hold on a second— allow me to clarify. While Panic disorders may mean that anxiety is here to stay - Anxiety is **treatable**, no matter how severe.

Entire books can be written (and have) about the treatments for anxiety and panic attacks. Many medications, meditative exercises, behavioral techniques, mindset adjustments, mantras, lifestyle changes, and so much more help people like me lead everyday lives. Some of these techniques, or even a combination of them, can treat anxiety and make it vanish into thin air for precious stretches of time.

A combination of these methods, mainly medication and mindset changes, have proved to work for *me* repeatedly, and during those moments of tranquility, I've grown immensely. Those very same panic attacks that constantly convinced me I was knocking on death's door have allowed me to understand myself and others on a deeper, more empathetic level. Reflecting on my moments of sheer terror, everything else in life seems like a piece of cake. My panic attacks have equipped me with the tools to help others navigate their feelings and get through whatever challenges they face, no matter how big or small. And when everything is okay, I can genuinely say that, at times, I'm thankful for what I've been through.

And then—another attack.

But John, that doesn't answer the big question. What is a panic attack? What does it feel like that so sets it apart from run-of-the-mill anxiety?

I am glad you asked, but truthfully, everyone struggles to put into words the outlandish thoughts and feelings that happen during an attack, so let me take a moment away from the scientifics, and instead focus on what matters – the feelings. Follow along:

Picture yourself sitting on your couch, eagerly watching the newest episode of *The Bachelorette.* You've been dying to see this episode because, according to the previews, your favorite contestant is about to grace the screen shirtless, and they're a total hottie.

At this moment, nothing can bring you down.

Then even though you live alone, you hear something. The front doorknob creaks, an eerie sound that reverberates through your bones. Someone—or something—is attempting to turn it ever so slowly. Fear takes hold of your heart, squeezing it mercilessly while an oppressive lump lodges itself in your throat. You want to dismiss the sound as your imagination running wild, but an unshakable unease gnaws at your every nerve. To confirm your safety, however, you slowly and carefully journey toward the door.

As you rise from the couch, your legs betray you, their strength reduced to nearly nothing. The deafening thuds of your heartbeat reverberate within the confined space of your skull. "Calm down," you whisper to yourself. "Everything is fine."

With each step you take, the panic intensifies. You're just a mere two feet from the door, staring at the door handle, and then—**bam!** The door bursts from the hinges.

Your mind reels in disbelief and terror, struggling to process the pandemonium that has erupted before you. You attempt to draw a breath and let loose a scream trapped within your constricted throat, but your voice is stolen. At that moment, you stand paralyzed, caught between fight and flight as time stands still but stretches infinitely all at once—an infinite void.

That moment right there - when the door bursts and you can't breathe, when you try to scream but the sound won't come out when you know you should run but you haven't the faintest idea what you're running from—*that* encapsulates the essence of a panic attack. Now, stretch out that feeling over five minutes, twenty minutes, or even a torturous four hours. That, my friend, is what a panic attack feels like.

However, during a panic attack, you likely won't have an intruder breaking into your home. The sound of the doorknob rattling might have been a fleeting "what if" thought that set your heart racing. The walk toward the door symbolizes the thoughts spiraling in your mind until they culminate in a moment of absolute terror - the burst of a door, triggering your fight-or-flight response. All this happens in response to a threat that may be entirely nonexistent.

Back to Science.

Interestingly, our brains react in strikingly similar ways in both scenarios. Regardless of whether your shirtless man on TV was interrupted by a home intruder or if your brain decided, for no apparent reason, to unleash a panic attack, the same cocktail of chemicals is released. A surge of adrenaline heightens your heart rate and body temperature. You break out into a sweat, and your muscles tense up. Your body flips the switch into fight-or-flight mode, desperate to escape. Nonsensical thoughts begin to orbit your mind and those "what if" scenarios morph into seemingly real threats you convince yourself of until it all ends.

Your brain *eventually* convinces you that the panic attack is over, that there was never any real danger, and your body gradually comes down from its heightened state.

Once it's all said and done, there's something of a panic attack hangover. After the adrenaline rush subsides, your body relaxes, finally freed from the gripping tension it endured. It's common to feel physically exhausted, with sore muscles and an overwhelming need to sleep.

In my case, I pee—a lot. Apparently, those are the muscles that calm down first for me.

Immediately after a panic attack, the trigger that set it off suddenly seems so minuscule. How could something so seemingly insignificant have caused such a monumental freakout? Did I genuinely consider jumping out the window during my meeting at work and running into the woods? (Yes, this one actually happened to me.)

Regardless, like finishing a long race, the aftermath for me is always followed by a feeling of total relaxation. Go figure. It isn't uncommon for me to fall asleep after an attack, even if I avoid the Xanax to get through it. I have found that it is crucial for me to embrace this hangover effect and take a moment to reflect. These are the moments when our minds find themselves most clear and rational. Don't let these moments simply pass you by.

So, let's recap and try one final time to answer this impossible question: What *exactly* is a panic attack? It's a chemical reaction to a fear that may or may not exist. It's far more complex than merely feeling scared or anxious. Panic attacks are one of the most terrifying experiences a person can go through, but they also make us stronger with each one we conquer. They are your episode of *The Bachelorette* interrupted. They are moments when our brains stop acting rationally and instead fill themselves with completely impossible and irrational considerations. And above all, panic attacks serve as a testament to how intricate and mysterious our brains are.

But, above all else, a Panic Attack is something that always ends, and you will *always* conquer. Promise.

"No amount of me trying to explain myself was doing any good.
I didn't even know what was going on inside of me,
so how could I have explained it to them?

Sierra D. Waters, Debbie.

2
My Soccer Ball Pillow

I've mentioned before that some people's anxiety can stem from irrational fears, and I'm a prime example of that. Many of my panic attacks seem to appear out of thin air like a bad magic trick. However, like me, many people who experience panic attacks also have very specific triggers.

I, for instance, am absolutely terrified of throwing up.

This trigger has dictated my every move my whole life. I have had times when I couldn't eat more than a few bites all at once because that feeling of being full triggered my worst nightmares: *what if I got sick?* I have had to avoid greasy food like the plague - That could make me sick. Lunchtime at school became a strategic operation. I had to sit near the door in case I suddenly felt queasy and needed to swiftly escape to throw up—or worse, if someone else threw up *in front* of me.

My fear escalated to the point where I had to leave school early one day, not because *I* was sick but because there was a rumor that Tim threw up outside his English class on the other side of the school. What if I had to walk that way later in the day or, heaven forbid, if I inhaled his germs and got sick myself? Yeah, no, thank you. I needed to go home.

This fear took on a life of its own as I grew through my younger years. While other kids were enjoying the simple pleasures of childhood, I was missing out due to this irrational fear. I avoided hamburgers for a solid eight years of my life simply because I once got sick after eating one before, and *what if* another hamburger makes me throw up again?

No macaroni, no root beer, nothing too colorful, and don't even get me started on oatmeal—it would all look disgusting if I happened to get sick after eating it.

Car rides became nightmarish journeys because I'm prone to motion sickness (of course I am). And what if it happened again? What if I threw up?

This fear of throwing up spiraled and spiraled, engulfing everything in its path like a black hole of terror. It morphed into a fear of food, a fear of going to friends' houses, a fear of school, a fear of cars—ultimately, a fear of life itself.

Let me tell you a story.

I was seven years old, visiting my doctor for a standard checkup. It was a sunny day, and my mom and I enjoyed some Burger King chicken fingers on the way there (but no fries for me. I never liked fries growing up). I felt fantastic as I entered the doctor's office, ready to conquer the world. I perused the children's magazines in the waiting room, which was always the highlight of my visits. I even charmed the nurses because I was a ladies' man in the making (little did I know, I was also gay, but that's a story for another time). I did feel a tad anxious when they took my blood pressure—the squeezing sensation wasn't exactly my cup of tea. But I put on a brave face for my hopefully future wife (the nurse).

Then came the moment of truth—time to get my weight. I stepped onto the scale, wearing nothing but my Pokémon tighty-whities, and the nurse read out my weight: **37 pounds**.

That number didn't faze me at the time. I basked in the glory of my 37 pounds of pure awesomeness. Little did I know, this was not "good news." I couldn't comprehend why being 37 pounds at seven was such a big deal then. I mean, everyone wants to be skinny, right?

The rest of the day passed by without a second thought. It wasn't until much later in life that I realized just how sick I was back then.

I didn't stop eating out of stubbornness. I stopped eating because fear gripped me tightly. I was afraid of eating and all the feelings it brought. I was severely underweight, and nothing seemed to bring my appetite back. I was forced to have protein shakes to cram in some calories, but it wasn't enough. My two older brothers wouldn't even let me take my shirt off in front of them because my body looked like a walking skeleton, and it freaked them out.

Believe it or not, that 37-pound weight measurement wasn't even the most shocking one I've encountered. Fast forward to age twelve, just a month before my thirteenth birthday—when my panic attacks had reached their climax. I was admitted to the mental ward of the children's hospital for a week when my attacks were at their worst. As I stepped onto the scale to be admitted, the nurse wrote down my weight: **55 pounds.**

Five years had passed since my weigh-in at the doctor's office, and during that time, I had gained a measly 18 pounds. Kids my age were going through growth spurts, eating food like ravenous beasts, and growing at a breakneck pace. Meanwhile, my body begged for nourishment, pleading with me to provide the desperately needed fuel. And yet, as much as my body begged, my mind fought back and would not allow myself to eat. Food was the enemy.

It's not like throwing up was even that common for me. As a kid, I hardly ever threw up. I had no reason to be scared because it rarely happened. I can vividly recall the only four times it happened before that weigh-in. That's it. And each time was before I was even seven years old.

Even more surprising, after my last puke experience at seven, it would be a whole thirteen years before I ever experienced another bout of vomiting - thirteen more years of that fear gripping my life.

So, why did this irrational fear of throwing up grip my life so tightly? That's a great question that I may never have the answer to. Even still, panic attacks related to this fear became a nightly ritual. Since I had only thrown up at night prior, the fear of throwing up always reached a peak as the sun set, when my fear of the fear itself would begin the attack. Ritualistically, I saw the skies go dark and began to panic, anticipating my nightly attack— a trigger without an actual trigger.

Panic attacks as a young kid are *very* confusing. If you think a home intruder is scary when they interrupt your beloved reality TV show, imagine that feeling multiplied tenfold in the heart and mind of a six-year-old wanting to watch Cartoon Network in peace. Children already struggle to comprehend and cope with intense emotions and anxiety. Well, panic attacks take those emotions to another stratosphere.

For me, a panic attack at that age consisted of a medley of symptoms. I would cry until my nose turned into a faucet, scream so loudly that my parents feared the neighbors might call child protective services, I would shake so violently that I burned more calories than I probably consumed that day. And I'd flail my arms so erratically that anyone within a ten-foot radius risked a bruise.

Now, at twenty-eight, only some of those symptoms persisted.

I scream less now.

Still, the fear of throwing up haunts me every day. What I carry with me *now* is over twenty years of learning how to cope and deal with this fear.

Most people have a safe space during panic attacks, and at that young age, the *bathroom* became my fortress. It was my sanctuary. If I needed to throw up, the logical solution was that the toilet must be the ideal place. Also, my irritable bowel syndrome would always flair during my attacks, so the bathroom was made for my attacks.

Babysitters, aunts, uncles, and even my father couldn't comprehend what caused these fears and why I couldn't simply shake them off. Fortunately, my mother, who also grew up with panic attacks, understood. She quickly became the person I relied on.

During those years, my full-blown panic attacks would stretch on for hours, full intensity from start to finish, occurring every single day without fail. I spent countless hours in the bathroom, wailing about the minimal but real possibility of vomiting. My brothers would grumble about not being able to focus on homework over my screaming, and my dad would raise the volume on the TV so he could hear Alex Trebek.

And there I would sit, in the bathroom, as I shook, teeth chattering, and screamed my way through the "what ifs" that loomed in the recesses of my mind.

And, every night, when the anxiety would finally exhaust me to the point of sleep, I would sprawl out on the cool, tiled floor of the bathroom, my mother gently stroking my back, whispering words of reassurance. I would rest my head on the seat of the toilet, using my favorite pillow at the time—an adorable white pillow shaped like a soccer ball—and every night, I would scream and cry myself to an exhausted sleep, waiting to throw up.

Even though every night, when all was said and done, I would manage to survive without throwing up, my certainty grew stronger that *one night* (probably the next) it would happen.

Let me be clear: This wasn't a case of neglect or a lack of effort to address the root issue. As you have read, I was no stranger to doctor's offices and had an arsenal of tools to get through these attacks. I repeated these techniques like a mantra during every attack, reminding myself what to do. I diligently took my medication (once I finally got some). And, when I wasn't in the throes of a panic attack, I was a genuinely happy kid.

But even with all these methods in place, I still spent more nights than I remember lying on the bathroom floor with my head on my soccer ball pillow.

To anyone reading this and resonating with my story, remember that your fears may feel overwhelming or irrational, but they do not define you. Sure, your worries may be crazy— maybe you're afraid of nothing during an attack—but that is okay. What matters is how you grow. Remember how important it is to be hopeful and resilient so that you too may grow from your experiences.

With patience, support, and a willingness to confront those fears, you will grow strong and be able to continue to win your war.

"Sometimes the people around you won't understand your journey. They don't need to, it's not for them."

Joubert Botha

3
A Day in the Life

E ven when I am doing well, anxiety is a daily battle for me. Sometimes, the battle is easy, like stopping a chihuahua from biting you. Sometimes, though, the anxiety is a big, muscly Great Dane with a mouth as strong as the jaws of life. And while my personal agenda changes daily, my anxiety dog follows its own agenda, which is almost always the same.

Every morning, when the dreams stop and I first wake, my first thought is always the same: *"How am I feeling today?"* In an instant, I analyze my whole body for unwelcome physical sensations and my entire mind for the same unwelcome thoughts. It is like I do a full-body sweep for anxiety before I let it find me first. Usually, this goes well, but sometimes I start my day first thing with an attack.

Regardless—and this part you will be mad at me for—the next step for me every day is one cup of regular coffee. I know: caffeine is the enemy of people like me. But I will tell you what: I do not like the mornings. My grumpy ass is entirely unpleasant until that coffee is finished. It's habitual, sure, but science is science, and this step is a non-negotiable science for me. If you spent one morning with me, you would agree.

Also, like many people, I always feel a tad nauseous when first waking up, and I can never force myself to eat breakfast. The thought of food in the morning repulses me. I feel sick if I try to eat.

Analyzing this tells me that it is all due to my fear of throwing up, and that if I eat, my stomach will settle and I will be okay. I know this is true because there are three things, for whatever reason, I can always convince myself to eat: apples, yogurt, and smoothies. No matter how nauseous I may be, these three breakfast foods are items I can eat every day.

Why don't I, you ask? Well, I always forget to buy more apples, and yogurt requires a spoon—not conducive to my morning commute. I am way too lazy to make my own smoothies, and not even Elon Musk can afford a daily morning smoothie from a smoothie shop. So instead, my breakfast is always just one cup of black coffee on an empty stomach, which leaves me feeling a bit jittery and angers my stomach just that much more.

This isn't too much of a big deal on workdays as I am usually distracted, and distraction is the best medicine when it comes to anxiety. On days off, though, I generally have lingering anxiety until lunchtime.

Lunchtime is another battle *every* day. Two significant factors come into play: before eating and after eating. Before eating, I need to convince myself *daily* that eating is okay. I may be starving, but unfortunately, my brain likes to confuse the feeling of starvation with the inevitability of throwing up. This starts a battle, usually short, where I convince myself that I just need food.

Then I finally eat, and after the first bite, my brain becomes completely convinced that the feelings I had were just hunger. You know that first bite of food when you were hungry just moments before— nothing beats that euphoria. So, in a manic moment of finally eating so many hours after waking, I shove my face with food. I do it compulsively every single day, even knowing the consequences.

And the consequence every day is a feeling of eating too much, too fast, where I am convinced again that I am going to throw up. This mini-anxiety episode usually does not last long, but it is a daily struggle, even in my best days.

Then, as long as I am medicated and in a good place, the next few hours are almost always calm. This is when I get my most work done on a workday or play the most hours of Zelda on a day off.

The next moment of anxiety comes around 5 pm every day, like clockwork. At this point, my afternoon is switching to nighttime. As the sun sets, my anxiety rises—it always has. There is something about evening that does this to me every day. It could be the spooky nature of the night—the setting of all horror stories. Or it could be from my nights with my soccer ball pillow. Either way, not a day goes by that this does not turn into a battle.

I ask myself the same questions at this time every day: How is my body feeling? Am I nauseous? Am I anxious? Do I feel like I will be?

I almost always answer these thoughts with distraction. Whether at this point, I am playing video games, having beers with friends, or even writing a book, distraction is my daily self-medication.

Self-medication comes in many forms. My self-medication comes in a relatively tame form, but the honest truth is that we all self-medicate in some way. We eat ice cream when we're sad or spend too much money when we're happy. We have caffeine every morning to wake up or take NyQuil to go to sleep. Self-medication can be very tame, but unfortunately, it is a dangerous path that can lead to negative life-changing addictions or other factors.

These distractions I force myself to have carry me straight to bed. Going to bed is hit or miss as well. Either I am tired and fall right asleep (the hope), or my anxiety surges anew and I spend the night wallowing on the couch or going for a few-mile-long walk. Either way, it ends the same—eventually, I fall asleep and do it all again.

Now, every day is unique. I have good days and bad days, just like everyone else. Sometimes my vices are replaced with spending time with friends, and sometimes (albeit rarely) I even make it to Denny's for breakfast.

My unfortunate reality is that even on the good days, there is a template that incorporates the things I try to avoid: my anxiety.

So, what do I do knowing this? Well, it sucks living with anxiety daily, but that is not the life lesson I have learned. Instead, I have learned to take in and appreciate the good for all its worth.

Enjoy the little things we all take for granted because sometimes the storm returns, and you forget just how good it can be.

In other words, remember how clearly you can breathe through your nostrils so that the next time you have a cold, you don't take that moment for granted.

"You don't have to control your thoughts.
You just have to stop letting them control you."

Dan Millman

4
The Panic Paradox

As I battled with panic attacks, one technique ingrained in me growing up was the power of rationalization - that is, to take a moment to focus on what I was feeling and thinking in the moment. In doing so, one could be able to rationalize things such as:

"Oh, I actually *can* breathe."

"What I am currently scared of is not real."

"Yes, there is a lump in my throat, but that is normal for an anxiety attack."

Or, even:

"Getting off this train because it's giving you anxiety would leave you stranded 600 miles from home, and it would still take a subsequent train or plane ride to get you home, which would only, in turn, result in more anxiety."

Believe it or not, these grounding thoughts are my way of returning to reality. I have to break down the anxiety, strip it of its power, and expose it for what it truly is: irrational. (And yes, I genuinely contemplated the idea of stranding myself in a foreign city with no plan and a dwindling bank account, all just to escape the feeling of being trapped on a train. Desperate times.)

Next, deep breaths. Ah, the glorious deep breaths. Inhale, feel the air filling your lungs. Notice the expansion, the life-giving oxygen saturating your body. Take a moment to truly feel what's happening in your hands and feet—those tingling sensations? They're just a quirky side effect of the anxiety attack. And as your heart races, feel each beat and contemplate why it's quickening. And guess what? Feel it slow down, too. You've got this.

Now, let me tell you, these grounding thoughts are a godsend. They have truly helped me regain control and navigate my way through the storm. Of course, firmly believing in them often takes a few repetitions and reminders, but they work. They are my lifeline.

Until they don't work.

"Pay attention to what's happening in your body," I'd whisper. "Understand why these sensations are occurring."

And so, I would take a deep breath and analyze my physical state. But then it hit me—I felt that crippling nausea, the lump in my throat, and I had to remind myself that these symptoms were common during anxiety. I'd tell myself, *Relax, it's just the anxiety making you queasy. It won't harm you.* Yet, a nagging thought persisted: *What if I still throw up?*

And just like that, the anxiety would surge again, perpetuating the vicious and self-perpetuating cycle. The side effects of my anxiety became my triggers, and no amount of logical reasoning could diminish the very real fear of vomiting that lurked within me.

DEEP BREATHS | 45

So far, throughout this book, we have covered a few things about myself and how they pertain to my anxiety, but let me recount a few important notes:

- I suffer from pretty extreme anxiety and panic attacks.
- Anxiety attacks cause physical feelings such as nausea.
- I am terrified of throwing up.

So, to further clarify, I'm scared of throwing up, which causes a panic attack, which makes me nauseous, and in turn makes me scared to throw up, which furthers my panic attack, and.....

You get the picture.

The side effects of my anxiety are my triggers, and no amount of acknowledging their harmless source reduces the risk they present. It isn't always as easy as reminding myself that the chest pain from my anxiety attack is not a heart attack and that a heart attack was not a possibility because, the nausea I feel still gives me the very real possibility of throwing up, which terrifies me to absolute hell.

This feedback loop is my biggest enemy in conquering my anxiety attacks. It requires more than just managing the anxiety itself. I have to find ways to address and alleviate the symptoms that accompany it.

Did you know that lightly sniffing isopropyl alcohol can almost instantly stop the feeling of nausea? I do.

Ginger tea, alcohol wipes, resting my head between my knees, and even prescription nausea medication have become standard supplements to all the anxiety tools I use to get through every panic attack.

Nowadays, I can't leave the house without my trusty Panic Attack Tool Kit (I should really trademark that). And you know what? It's perfectly okay. What works for one person may only work for one person. We all have unique struggles and require personalized approaches to tackle them. Mine just happens to be a bag of ways to combat nausea.

Often, I found myself discouraged by the complexities of my "Panic Paradox"—the notion that my anxiety feeds on itself, perpetuating a never-ending cycle of anxiety. My panic attacks would always be worse than others, so I would never get better at handling them.

But I was wrong. With each panic attack, I have learned something new about myself. I have discovered what tools and techniques work best for me. Sure, it means adding a few more gadgets to my Panic Attack Tool Kit, but that's okay.

During this ongoing journey, I've come to realize that anxiety is not my enemy. It's a part of my story, a chapter in the book of my life (or the whole book in this case). And as I continue to navigate through the twists and turns, I'm finding strength I never knew I had. Anxiety has forced me to confront my fears head-on, push beyond my comfort zone, and embrace the beauty of resilience and personal growth.

Sometimes, when I find myself caught in the whirlwind of anxiety, I seek solace in the company of others who understand.

It's comforting to know that I'm not alone in this battle. Sharing our stories, listening to the experiences of fellow anxious folk, and offering support creates a sense of community and reminds us that we're in this together. And that, together, we can overcome the challenges that anxiety throws our way.

So, my fellow anxiety enjoyers, let's embrace the journey of self-discovery armed with our unique sets of coping mechanisms. And who knows, maybe someday we'll gather around at an anxiety support group meeting, sharing tales of our odd remedies and unconventional tools, all while offering support and understanding.

If you are entangled in your own Panic Paradox, don't limit yourself to the recommended tools and strategies. Explore, experiment, and find those additional tools that resonate with you. Your anxiety project may require a few extra tools from the Home Depot of Life, but trust me, it's worth it. There is always room for growth, learning, and adaptability when it comes to panic attacks.

No matter how bad your panic, or how strong the paradoxical side effects, remember: Keep calm, carry on, remember you are not alone, and never forget to pack your own Panic Attack Tool Kit.

You are not alone

The following is a list of famous people from current times and throughout history who have come out and said that they too also suffer(ed) from panic attacks and/or anxiety.

1. Oprah Winfrey
2. Adele
3. Kim Kardashian
4. Kristen Bell
5. Emma Stone
6. Megan Thee Stallion
7. Jonah Hill
8. Kendall Jenner
9. Prince Harry
10. Lady Gaga
11. Ariana Grande
12. Whoopi Goldberg
13. Stephen Colbert
14. Chris Evans
15. Ryan Reynolds
16. Princess Diana
17. David Bowie

18. Johnny Depp

19. Sigmund Freud

20. Edvard Munch (which explains his famous painting, *The Scream*)

21. Michael Phelps

22. Gina Rodriguez

23. Carson Daly

24. Missy Elliot

25. Jennifer Lopez

26. Leonardo DiCaprio

27. Hugh Grant

28. Harry Styles

29. Amanda Seyfried

30. John Mayer

31. Caitlyn Jenner

32. Lizzo

33. Abraham Lincoln

And so many more.

5
The Spongebob Squarepants Movie

I was born in 1995, which might seem young to some and too old to be cool to others, but what truly matters is that when *The SpongeBob Squarepants Movie* hit theaters in November 2004, I was nine years old, the perfect age for such a film. I was brimming with excitement for that animated masterpiece in Bikini Bottom.

But first, let's rewind a bit. As a child of the early 2000s, we didn't identify ourselves by our sexual preferences or gender identities. No, no, we had a more crucial identity to uphold—whether we were Nickelodeon, Disney Channel, or Cartoon Network kids. It was like factions in the great war of cartoons (which, by the way, were at their peak during that time). And let me tell you, I was a die-hard member of Team Cartoon Network.

But amid this great war, a united front united all kids across America and beyond. No matter, if you belonged to Team Nickelodeon or not, every single one of us *was* a SpongeBob Kid (and likely still is).

I vividly recall those school days when our librarian would wheel in that clunky CRT television on the iconic TV cart and we would sit, me and my fellow students, traversing the vibrant

Jellyfish Fields or participating in The Fry Cook Games, all in the company of SpongeBob and his friends together.

SpongeBob Birthday Parties? *Check.* SpongeBob Pajamas? *Check.* SpongeBob Halloween costumes? *Triple check.* It was a SpongeBob extravaganza, saturating every nook and cranny of our young lives.

So, to a wide-eyed nine-year-old in 2004, the release of *The Spongebob Squarepants Movie* was *the* most exciting thing our little minds had ever waited for.

For perspective, It's kind of like how, as a twenty-year-old homosexual, I was excited beyond belief to witness the one and only Lady Gaga performing at the 2017 Pepsi Super Bowl Halftime Show.

All of this to say, when it came time to finally watch the movie, *nothing* could bring me down.

But here's the twist: Something *would* manage to bring down my SpongeBob-fueled euphoria that fateful day. And if you've been paying attention, you can probably guess what it was.

Movies possess a mystical power. They stick with you, influence you, and shape you—especially when you're young and impressionable. A movie, for whatever reason, when watched at the right age, can be the cause of a lifetime of influence.

Sometimes, these influences are positive. Perhaps, at the young age of seven, you witnessed Luke Skywalker single handedly save the galaxy from imminent destruction, and that inspired you to become a force of good in the world. Or *Interstellar* may have fueled your early passion for aerospace engineering, leading you to design rocket ships fifteen years later.

The positive impacts of movies are boundless. Unfortunately, though, so are the negative ones.

Take *Signs*, for example. After watching M. Night Shyamalan's film, I couldn't peek out of a window without envisioning spiky aliens lurking outside. And the Ringwraiths from *The Lord of the Rings* visited me in a recurring nightmare for months on end.

Even my mom had a similar experience as a kid. Since her childhood viewing of *The Wizard of Oz*, she has been haunted to this day. Just hearing the iconic music triggers her heart to race. And honestly, I get it—almost everything (with the exception of Toto) is terrifying in that film.

However, the night of *The SpongeBob Squarepants Movie* was not ruined for me by an impression it made that night. No, I was not scared of the movie starring the happiest sponge on the ocean floor. The culprit responsible for ruining that night was none other than the 2004 blockbuster hit *The Day After Tomorrow*.

In case you're unfamiliar, this film portrays a series of catastrophic weather events leading to the end of humanity and life as we know it. Perfect movie material for an eight-year-old riddled with anxiety.

For months after watching that disaster flick, not a single rainy day went by without me convincing myself that our world was on the brink of destruction. I had the receptionist at my mother's workplace practically on speed dial, crying and begging to be transferred to my mom's cubicle phone whenever thunderstorms rumbled through the skies.

Movie theatres also became a no-go zone for me as a kid, likely induced by the loud-noise phobia of the thunder itself. So, for my inaugural viewing of *The SpongeBob Squarepants Movie*, I skipped the theatre release and instead planned a sleepover at my close friend's house on the day of the DVD release. We had the whole day planned to be the best day ever, and when the sun would fall, we would make the best popcorn, gather the best snacks, and watch the movie that we had been dying to see. And that is precisely what happened. Trampoline time during the day, getting excited for the movie, pool time where we pretended to be the Bikini Bottom bunch ourselves, and the coolest blanket fort ever constructed was in place and ready as the DVD slid into the DVD player. Two nine-year-old kids with the biggest smiles on their faces as the movie began to roll, and then—it thundered.

In an instant, Little John's radiant smile vanished. The world *was* ending, life as he knew it crumbling to pieces. Sure, little John was nestled in the most incredible blanket fort ever constructed, and the movie he had eagerly anticipated had just started playing. But this couldn't possibly be how he died!

Although close, my friend in the cool pillow fort had no idea about my panic attacks, and I was not about to look uncool in front of him. So, I did what I had to do—I swallowed my fear, forced my attention onto the movie, and hoped for a distraction to save the day.

The Krusty Krab was unveiling a Krusty Krab 2? Patrick was showcasing his flag-waving skills with his butt? The movie was hilarious, and everything should have been fine.

Then, more thunder.

And with each deafening roar, I became more and more sure—the world was unequivocally ending. I wouldn't have a chance to say goodbye to my loved ones. What would the cataclysmic storm that spelled our doom feel like? What does dying feel like?

The frantic thoughts were racing through my nine-year-old brain as I reluctantly embraced my impending fate. Not even "Goofy Goober Rock" could rescue me at that point.

Before I knew it, I was engulfed in a full-fledged panic attack. I began shaking, sobbing, and screaming. My friend's mom rushed in, confused by the chaos that had unfolded before her eyes. Kids get scared during thunderstorms all the time, but this was a reaction of an entirely different magnitude.

My friend seemed more annoyed than concerned about our failed movie night. He kept pestering me, asking if I was done panicking so we could find out if SpongeBob and Patrick would ever make it to Shell City.

I couldn't do it. I didn't make it through the movie, and my mom had to rescue me, braving the ongoing thunderstorm to drive a quarter of a mile between our houses and escort me home. The panic attack wouldn't stop after returning home either, even though the storm soon did.

That incident changed the dynamic of my friendship with that particular friend. Things never returned to normal, and we drifted apart soon after. Thus, my first attempt at a sleepover at a friend's house ended in disappointment, and it would be years before I mustered the courage and successfully completed my first sleepover.

However, *I am* proud to announce that I eventually conquered *The SpongeBob Squarepants Movie.*

Also, now, it takes a genuinely cataclysmic storm to persuade me that the world is on its last legs.

Progress.

"Don't be ashamed of your story. It will inspire others."

Unknown

6
To Be Seen

Your first panic attack is undeniably terrifying. So is your fifth, tenth, or thousandth. And even at such high numbers, each one can feel worse than the last. They can haunt you for years, showing up at the most inconvenient times like an uninvited guest who overstays their welcome. And trust me, I've had my fair share of unwelcome visitors.

Having panic attacks at a young age made everything feel even scarier. As kids, we're already prone to being scared of things that adults find laughable. We watch horror movies and run screaming from the room, only to giggle about our reactions later in life. But what if the fear persists? What if it lingers and refuses to dissipate, leaving you in a state of perpetual anxiety? That was my reality.

Sure, I was afraid of throwing up, which caused a majority of my attacks. I feared the world ending, which accounted for quite a few more. I was afraid of so much and all that fear caused almost every single attack. Almost.

But there were times when panic attacks struck without warning, without any discernible cause. It was like being caught in a storm without a cloud in sight. Confusing doesn't even begin to describe it, especially for a young mind trying to make sense of it all.

"What are you even afraid of?"

A question so simple I would be asked during these attacks. What are you afraid of? Why are you crying? Why *are* you shaking?

"I don't know," I would weep in defeat. How could I not know what I was afraid of, but be reacting in such a major way?

Many people struggled to understand. My father, for instance, never understood why I couldn't just snap out of it. Aunts, uncles, and babysitters were equally confused, unsure of what the hell to do to comfort a child who seemed to be unraveling without a cause. I was surrounded by confusion, my own and that of all those who cared about me—except for one person: my mom.

When I would cry to my mom, terrified and snot running down my face from who knows what, she would look me in the eyes and tell me she understood exactly what I meant and was going through. These simple words would ground me time and time again if even just a little.

I felt seen.

It probably helped that she has had panic attacks too. I don't know too much about how biology works, but I am pretty sure I can thank my sweet mother for passing these puppies down to me genetically. (And remember the IBS? That one was my dad.) My mom suffered panic attacks her whole life, and that understanding she brought was so important to me as I began going through and navigating my own crazy times. I had her, and that made it so much better. I was so lucky to have her as I navigated that unchartable sea.

But my mother's journey was not as easy. She grew up in a time when mental health wasn't talked about. When it was swept under the rug or treated as an inconvenience rather than a genuine concern. Her parents didn't believe in panic attacks and dismissed them with a simple, "Just get over it." It took her years to find solace and validation, to feel truly seen for the first time.

I can't help but be grateful for our progress as a society since then. Today, mental health is a topic of discussion and a vital part of our culture. We're breaking down the barriers, smashing the stigma, and supporting countless people who face their own battles. More and more children and adults are finding the support systems they deserve.

But the truth remains: too many people still suffer in silence. Too many are forced to bury their emotions and navigate the labyrinth of fear alone. So many people grapple with the confusion of being terrified of nothing, and their cries for understanding often go unheard.

That's why I'm here, sharing these stories from my life. I want to create a space where you, the reader, can find solace and recognition. You are not alone. What you're going through is significant and real, even if it feels like you're afraid of nothing at all. Even if nobody understands you, let these pages be your friend.

Society has come a long way in acknowledging anxiety and mental health. It is essential to spread this awareness so that others may feel that they are not alone.

And sometimes, that is all you need – someone to just simply say, "I get it, I know what you are going through."

So - Within these words, within these narratives, and within this world, you are seen.

A Poem

Look at yourself.
Look in that mirror right in front of you.
Stare yourself in the eyes.
It's time for a pep talk — you **need** to get through this.

What are you going to do otherwise?
Run? You can't.
You're on an airplane.
And you didn't pack a parachute.

Five more hours. Just five more hours.
You promised yourself you wouldn't let your panic attacks
keep you from traveling.
You promised yourself you would fight through it no matter what.
You promised.

You are **okay**.
You are **strong.**
You are **capable.**
You can do this.

7
New fears,
or more of the same?

I'm sure you could guess this about me, but I am afraid of a lot of things. Yeah, I like to put on a brave face, but truth be told, I'm a scaredy cat.

On the laundry list of fears I own, another incredibly strong fear, is flying. Airplanes? They freak me out, man. I mean, the takeoff, the landing, turbulence? Everything about flying sends me into a full-blown panic attack.

Not too long ago, I had to take a flight from Chicago to Boston. Short and smooth, no real need for anxiety.

I'm sorry. Have you met me? I spent the entire flight shaking like a leaf. At one point, I even looked over and saw the man next to me texting a friend: "This guy next to me can't stop shaking and it's pissing me off. Probably needs heroin or something." Heroin! He thought my panic attack was heroin withdrawal.

The day of that flight (or any for that matter) was a whole frickin' ordeal. It started with me forcing food down my throat because, you know, an empty stomach and a turbulent plane don't exactly go hand in hand. And coffee? Oh yeah, I got to have my morning fuel, but not too much 'cause it'll only amp up the anxiety.

Then comes the strategic planning of my Dramamine dosage. Take it too soon, and I'll be a zombie throughout the day. Take it too late, and I might puke my guts out on the plane. Luckily this dosage doubles as my relaxant.

Now, traveling is always a reason for a little liquid celebration, but alcohol and Dramamine don't mix. Plus, what if I grab a beer at the airport, and it makes me dizzy during takeoff? That'd make me sick. But hey, one beer could calm my nerves, right?

So, I (mostly) skip the beer and make my way to the gate. That's when I find a seat, plop myself down, and start contemplating all the ways things could go wrong. I stare out the gate window at that monstrous metal contraption I'll soon be locked inside, and for a brief moment, I consider if it's too late to bail.

Boarding groups get called, and deep down, I secretly hope they'll forget mine and I'll get to escape the whole airport scene. Who needs to travel, right?

But of course, they never forget my boarding group (the nerve of some people), and I reluctantly shuffle my way onto the plane. This is where the fun begins. The moment I cross that threshold, my heart kicks into overdrive, threatening to pop out of my throat. The humming of the plane motors becomes a ringing hum within my own mind, synchronizing with my increasing heartrate and drowning out all other sounds. "Focus on finding your seat," I chant to myself, hoping it'll keep me somewhat sane. Sometimes, the flight attendants notice my anxiety and give my shoulder a reassuring rub as I pass. Sometimes the captains stand out of the cockpit and greet the boarding people and kids. I always look at them and wonder what kind of crazy person would choose that career, and why the heck are they only handing out those cool plastic wings to the little ones?

Anyway, next, I find my seat. This is a bit tricky. You see, I can't have a window seat, because then I am trapped. But a window seat would be better so I can look out the window and avoid being disoriented. Still, I look for an aisle seat. Aisle seats are best, so I can always get up and run should I need to. The only thing is, the man in the window seat better keep that damn window open, so I don't get disoriented.

The seatbelt needs to be tied, and the feeling of that thing wrapped around my waist constricts me like a snake. It traps me further, and binds me to my seat, which is not the place I want to be.

As the plane moves, the motors hum louder and tease the inevitable takeoff, which is the worst part. We move, and through glimpses out the windows, I am able to see that we finally pull onto the runway. My heartbeat is now so loud it threatens blowing out my eardrums, and my hands become a pool of sweat gripping the seat.

The engines roar, and the plane accelerates so quickly that I become glued to the back of my seat. The feeling reinforces the feeling of being weighed down and trapped and perpetuates the anxiety attack. As the plane climbs, so does my anxiety, despite the medication in my system. And just as the plane evens out, my anxiety plateaus, only to come down again with the plane, better only when my feet are safely on the ground, and I am free to go where I please.

Flying on planes, for me, is a mess. But through reflection I have noticed something about my fear of planes—it's not a fear of planes. Nope, it's a tangled mess of all my other fears bundled up into one terrifying package.

What if I need to throw up on the plane? What if someone else needs to throw up on the plane? Turning makes me dizzy, and the second the doors shut I feel trapped. I need to get out, what if I need to get out? Can planes crash? Will my world end? Why does the altitude make me feel funny? G-forces? No thank you.

It's never been just about the plane itself. It's about all the fears it contains, and the somatic symptoms I convince myself are real.

It's a *plane* ol' Panic Paradox again (I am proud of that pun thank you very much).

And let me tell you, this relationship between me and anxiety is a wild real rollercoaster. Moments like these make me realize that it's not about fear creating more fear. No, it's about each fear intertwining and amplifying each other, creating one big scary monster.

So, logistically speaking, the answer is simple: unpack each fear individually. And for many, that works like a charm. Let's start with the feeling of being trapped. Well, guess what? You don't need to escape 'cause you're perfectly fine. Fear of dying? Hey, planes rarely crash, and the odds of survival are in our favor—besides, you drive every day and that is *far* more dangerous. Fear of puking? I've got my trusty Dramamine, and the chances of barfing in the plane are as likely as on solid ground. And hey, they even provide those handy-dandy barf bags!

It should be easy, but for me, it's a one-way ticket to a spiral of "what if?" questions, compounding my fears even more. It's like smashing trash down to make more room instead of just taking it out. Yeah, it shrinks, but it's still there, compressed and lurking.

So, am I stuck on the ground? No. I do get on planes, and I do fly. How do I do it may you ask? Well, I would be delighted to tell you.

To get through flights, I bring to the front of my mind the 1999, twenty-five-year-running, one-thousand-plus-chapter, Japanese anime and manga titled, *One Piece.*

Literally, that's what I do. It's that easy. Let me explain:

One Piece follows the story of a courageous, and carefree pirate named Luffy. Luffy is a man who can stretch as if his body were made of rubber, and he sails the open seas to find the world's most coveted treasure: the One Piece.

Not following? Stick with me. You see, to gain his stretching power, Luffy had to give up the ability to swim. A pirate who can't swim presents a problem. If that were me in the One-Piece world, I would have an easy solution to that issue. Can't swim? Don't get on a boat.

But no, Luffy is fearless. He doesn't just sail the regular seas with his crew. No, he goes for the riskiest, most dangerous routes, all while sitting cross-legged on the figurehead of the ship, one slip of the butt away from potential death.

Now, you're probably wondering, *John, how the heck does thinking about this swimless pirate help you fly?*

To that I say, "Stop interrupting me. I'm getting there."

While there are lessons to be learned from Luffy's fearless exploits, there's one specific adventure I want to share with you.

One of the islands Luffy and his crew needed to get to was in the sky. To reach this island, Luffy and his crew needed to ride a geyser-like current that shot them miles through the sky. With the front of the ship facing the sun, they climbed until they could not see the ground below them.

The crew's reaction, much like my own on a plane, was that of absolute terror. Death was imminent.

But you know what? During that hair-raising journey, Luffy, the man most likely to meet a tragic end, continued to have fun as the ship climbed, all while baring a smile plastered on his face as he laughed and enjoyed the ride.

And that, my friend, is the big lesson right there. "Don't take life too seriously,"

Or maybe it's, "Be not afraid, but smile at the things that should fear you."

Or, maybe still the lesson is, "If you are a pirate that can't swim, do it anyway and have fun while you do it"

Regardless, visualizing the fearlessness of this fictional character has turned into a talisman that I carry to persevere. This helps during flights, but also in my every day. Bringing to mind anyone who uses their strength, either mental or physical, can carry you through moments of your own weakness. Empathizing with others and convincing yourself "If they can do it, so can I" is a powerful way to get through each battle.

Fear breeds fear - it is a fact of life. But with the right mindset, any fear no matter how compounded is conquerable. And, remember, if you find yourself flying through the air and afraid you will die, bring to mind a person of inspiration and remember: it is always easier to smile and just enjoy the ride.

"The only way out of the labyrinth of
suffering is to forgive."

John Green

8
Social Butterflies

I don't like meeting new people.

If you are reading this book and happen to know me personally, you might be surprised by this. There is even a story my mom tells far too often that really contradicts this statement.

Picture little third grade me, overflowing with confidence and a big mouth like no other. I was the coolest, and I needed to tell everyone. Forget going by John. I was Johnny - with an "h" for extra coolness.

I talked *a lot*. That never made my teacher's job very easy. This was especially true for my third-grade teacher. She tried everything to keep me down. First, she sat me next to the silent student—you know the one. Sure enough, within a week, he started talking more than me.

Next, she moved me next to an exchange student from Venezuela who didn't speak a lick of English. And you know what happened? Yep, she was speaking English within a week.

I, a third grader, outshined the ESL teacher.

There was nowhere in the classroom she could move me to keep me quiet. Left knowing that, she decided to place a square of duct tape on the floor, forming my very own desk island. I was to sit in that desk, and I was not allowed out of the square of tape unless I first asked—a true punishment.

Well, I think she thought it was a punishment, but I loved my island.

So, yes, as a kid, I loved talking and meeting new people—maybe a little too much. But as I grew older, that comfort disappeared, fading into the background. Nowadays, the thought of social gatherings or having to introduce myself is about as appealing as accidentally going to school in your underwear—a nightmare.

Of course, I don't exactly express these feelings to people. After all, even given these circumstances, I *do* consider myself a people person. In my day job, I interact directly with the public, and truth be told, I wouldn't have it any other way. I still love to talk—no surprise there.

However, there's an undeniable anxiety that comes with meeting new people, a shared experience for many, and a very real one for me. Even in my daily work, the thought of meeting new people always makes my stomach turn and my hands sweat.

When anxiety becomes your everyday sidekick, it casts a gloomy, anxious shadow over different aspects of your life. Mundane tasks suddenly become daunting challenges that must be conquered. The same is for work. A meeting with a client may exhaust me of all energy as that anxious storm has darkened my day.

As I grew older and away from my chatty youth, my anxiety took up residence in the depths of my mind, infiltrating my thoughts and influencing my entire mindset. The more obvious fears that I have discussed simply became worse: the dread of eating, the constant fear of throwing up, or the nagging sense that the world was on the brink of apocalyptic disaster.

However, my subconscious voice, loud and unmistakable yet still a silent assassin, loved to shout over the fence to its neighbor, my conscious mind. These thoughts were never anything I could hear in the moment, but each of these times, my anxiety would deepen. It's like my subconscious mind was a little angry chihuahua that just wanted to see me burn and would gnaw at me every chance it got.

Did you really say that?

Those people over there are whispering—*are they making fun of you?*

You smiled, and nobody else did. Everyone must think you're weird.

This relentless voice, or restless and oh-so-angry chihuahua of my subconscious mind, began whispering sweet, tormenting nothings that slowly poisoned my social life.

And let me tell you, I despise the idea of anxiety controlling my life.

So, I compensated. Throughout my middle-school years, I became the class clown, *determined* to make everyone like me. Compensation meant going too far a lot of the time, however, and I spent most of my middle-school years in detention or suspension.

Girlfriends became a must because, without them, I felt like a nobody. And even though it was in eighth grade that I realized that I liked boys, I continued dating girls until after high school just because image became an obsession, and being gay was not cool yet at the time. It wasn't that I didn't like these girls or that I used them—I truly fell in love. It was just that I was not complete. Most importantly though, my outward appearance and the opinions others had of me became crucial to my incredibly fragile self-worth.

It took a considerable amount of time and effort to locate that tiny voice in my head and silence it. However, even with the voice hushed, the damage it had done proved challenging to overcome—something I still work on every day.

Anxiety always finds new ways to show its teeth, leaving *you* to discover its many faces at every turn. But you know what? Despite the persistence of my anxiety, I've managed to grow and continue growing. I've learned to analyze when it tries to take control, and, through maturing, I no longer compensate after realizing how anxiety negatively affects me, but rather accept and flourish—and work on reversing that damage every day.

The anxiety may be here to stay; however, its damage is never permanent.

But, as of now, I still hate meeting new people.

"The only thing we have to fear is fear itself."

Franklin D. Roosevelt

9
"911. What's Your Emergency?"

At twelve-years and eleven-months old, my panic attacks had become so bad that I was admitted to the mental hospital for a hands-on evaluation. The eleven months in my age is important—not because every preteen counts down the months to their birthday. But because the fact that I was not yet a teenager, I was put with the younger children, and boy, did I not fit in.

Picture me, nearly thirteen, and as discussed, under 60 pounds, simply dealing with panic attacks, meanwhile I was surrounding by children who had severe depression, committed crimes, attempted suicide, or in one case, attempted homicide against their bus driver.

As I spent my week in that hospital and cried myself to sleep, I would ask myself, *Why the hell am I here?* But then I would convince myself that maybe I *am* a freak or a weirdo. In the end, I would always decide: "I don't belong here." (That one was for all you Radiohead fans.)

However, I had no idea that my time in that hospital would save my life.

This book is mostly a happy one, so I will skip the dark stories of that time and jump ahead to how it ended: my final psychiatric evaluation.

It was the end of my stay. They had collected all the data they needed, and I had collected a spicy chicken wrap from Wendy's every day when my mom would visit.

This day, I was to sit in a small room and wait for the psychiatrist. I had met many doctors and nurses and expected someone similar to arrive as the door opened. However, in walked a man, likely about three-hundred years old, who looked like if he was not yet dead—time was of the essence. That is all to say: he was very, *very* old.

They say old people are wise, that they have seen many things. Turtles are always the wise sage in animated films.

Well, this man was the Master Oogway of panic attacks. He was a panic attack specialist, and at three-hundred years old, he had seen many, many attacks.

He was the first man who finally recognized me for who I was. Someone who recognized my panic anxiety disorder, acknowledged my attacks for what they were, and most importantly, prescribed me the medication I needed to finally pull myself out of attacks when they finally came. He also diagnosed me with my Somatic Symptoms Disorder, which essentially can cause emotional distress to inflict physical symptoms. A lot of people experience this to a degree, but for me, it's engrained.

Oh, and did I mention? He said my attacks had been the worst he'd ever seen. This three-hundred-year-old specialist who had seen it all had never met a twelve-year and eleven-month boy like me.

You don't want a wise old turtle to tell you that.

But he did save my life. I made it out of that hospital homicide free, and from that day forward my life began to climb.

*   *   *

So, I mentioned that Somatic Symptom Disorder? Well, since that day, I have found myself back in the hospital a *small* but mighty handful more times—always for physical symptoms, rarely for anything more than a mental cause.

One time, pain in my nether region sent me to the hospital, as it was so bad I thought I had torn something. Not the area you really want a tear.

During that visit, a young nurse in training had to give her very first ultrasound. I hope she didn't give up on nursing school after that *experience*.

Kidney pain has sent me more than once. Once I'm convinced that my kidneys hurt, over time that pain can grow, somatically, in my head until it is unbearable.

Vertigo, headaches, stomach pain, you name it, I have been to the ER for it. And what becomes so frustrating is that to rule out these physical possibilities, doctors are forced to do *all* the tests.

And when the tests are complete, and everything comes back fine, I am left with no diagnosis and a long ride home as I battle with the realization that it was all in my head. The walk of shame, on a whole different level.

Hypochondria and Somatic Symptoms Disorder are very similar—a thought you may have already had. Just like someone with hypochondria, I obsess about my health. What sets it apart is that the symptoms I feel, are very real symptoms, but tests cannot find a cause.

And I know, not everyone has Somatic Symptoms Disorder, but many of us with anxiety have gone through this same journey. Often, that very first panic attack ends with a trip to the ER, so they can tell you that it's not a heart attack and Xanax will be the preferred treatment over a heart transplant. I have read statistics that over a million visits to the ER every year are anxiety related.

So despite Radiohead's opinion, we are not freaks or weirdos. We are in a very common majority. Understanding that has helped me try to treat anxiety first before spiraling into believing I am dying, and I suggest everyone with anxiety saves their money and does the same before calling 911.

And if all else fails, do what I do: make friends with the nurses.

"Mental health is not just the absence of mental illness.
It's about emotional, psychological, and social well-being."

Unknown

10
It Wasn't Always Bad

My times of intense anxiety come and go in waves. There have been years when I had panic attacks every day, and later years when I had no attacks at all. Never panic free, but free from full-blown attacks.

After my time in the hospital with that wise old turtle, and finding the right medication, I reached one of those periods of relief. Specifically, during high school, I had very few full-blown attacks. My overwhelming storm of anxiety had diminished to a more mist-like weather—a manageable level.

I owe a great deal of this improvement to the medication I was taking. Medication truly saved my life. If you fear taking medication, just know that when used correctly, it has the power to completely bring you back to reality and make you feel normal again. It has for me and many others.

Pills *can* be cool.

In addition to medication, many lifestyle changes can help with anxiety as well. You've probably heard it all. Improving diet, practicing meditation and yoga, engaging in breathing exercises, and most importantly, exercising regularly can reduce the frequency and severity of attacks. Deep breaths, I know.

To be honest, I used to dismiss cognitive approaches of reducing anxiety for a long time. They never worked for me before I started taking medication, and that worked so well that I didn't see the need to try anything else. Breathing techniques seemed like something out of Gwenyth Paltrow's GOOP (which was not yet a thing), and I wanted nothing to do with them.

Although, throughout high school, I was a varsity runner. When I started running, I never intended it to help with my anxiety; it didn't even cross my mind. I decided to join cross country for two reasons: I was in a new school and needed new friends, and one of the few friends I had made told me I should, so I did.

Little did I know that running would become incredibly therapeutic for me. The camaraderie of running with friends during practice always lifted my spirits. Practices in the rain where we would sing Lady Gaga and slide down hills would put me in a better place immediately. After completing a run, I always would experience a euphoric runner's high that made me feel invincible. Setting a new personal record in a race made me feel on top of the world.

Most importantly, exercise was doing wonders for my mental health chemically. I know, I know: "Running sucks." But for me, it was the best thing that had ever happened to me at the time. Of course, during a race or around mile three, you wouldn't hear me saying that, but looking back, it had a profound impact on my well-being.

Throughout that time, I was able to attend events, make numerous new friends, and even stay over at friends' houses—something, as I have discussed, was before impossible. Something as simple as going to a high school football game or school dance had been off-limits for me for a long time, but now I found myself attending such things *regularly.*

The reduction in my anxiety also allowed me to approach life from a different perspective. No longer did I feel the need to compensate for my anxiety by acting out. Instead, I embraced friendship with compassion and humor. Being funny can truly win friends—although only when you're not being a jerk about it. (I'm talking you, middle school me.)

I was heavily involved in film class for my four years of high school and hosted the daily news every morning for the entire school. The anxious person I used to be sat in front of a camera every day.

Me—on camera with (mostly) no nerves.

I became a completely different person from who I had ever been before.

Of course, I can't guarantee that exercise alone was responsible for this transformation. I was on the right medication and my mind and body were changing. Plus, I surrounded myself with people, some very important teachers who are still important to me, and a few new friends who would later become people I would spend my whole life connected to. All these factors combined led me to where I was during those years.

Now, as I continue to experience ups and downs, I remember that there will be more periods in my life, where the storm settles. I will have times when full-blown attacks are nothing but a memory, and during those times, it will be easy to take things for granted and forget how bad it can get. So, instead, I use calmer periods to learn and grow, preparing myself for the next wave. Anxiety comes and goes in waves, and with each wave, I prepare more and more for the next.

And if worst comes to worst, I guess I can go for a run.

The seven things I hate about panic attacks

1. Feeling like I can't catch my breath.
2. When a bad attack makes me scream and cry.
3. How they have, at many times, controlled my life.
4. Feeling like I need to run but having nowhere to go.
5. Some of my favorite things in life bring them on.
6. That one of the side effects of panic attacks is also one of my biggest triggers.
7. That every time, they feel like they will never end.

The seven things I love about panic attacks

1. They have taught me compassion and understanding.
2. When they are over, it can be fun to look back and laugh at how irrational you were.
3. Shaking violently *must* burn calories, right?
4. I have been able to help other people get through their own attacks, only because I have gone through them myself.
5. They make other hardships not so bad.
6. The times I actually exercise to get rid of them.
7. They always do end.

11
Daddio

It has been three months since the last time I talked to my dad.

I know. I should call him, but he could reach out to me too. That's how our relationship has always been. We can go weeks or even months without speaking, but when we do reconnect, it's as if no time has passed at all. I will call him soon.

The last time I saw my dad was during Christmas. It was a bittersweet gathering because my mom's sister had recently been diagnosed with leukemia, and we all knew it could potentially be our last holiday season together with her. So, the entire family came together, including my father and his girlfriend. Being reunited with my whole family and celebrating a holiday with both my mom and dad present for the first time in ages felt good.

However, my father couldn't stay for long.

But before I continue, excuse me for a moment. My phone is ringing. Why is my mom calling me this late?

"Hello?"

"Hi, John. Are you alone right now?"

"No, why? Is everything okay?"

"Can you sit down? I have something to tell you.

"Okay, okay, I'm sitting down. What's going on?"

"It's Daddy. He was in an accident, and... he didn't make it."

*   *   *

It has been five years since that night.

My dad was always a real joker. He was known for his sense of humor, even if it *was* somewhat unconventional. The same man who loved me dearly was the one who taught me that "dipshit" and "dumbass" could be terms of endearment. And he was funny right up until the day he passed away. The accident that took him away from us so suddenly five years ago was a prank gone wrong at his workplace—playing pranks right up until the end.

My dad was never very good with my panic attacks. I like to think it was because he has never dealt with a panic attack. His best way of handling things was, "Get over it" or "Let's just call your mom."

I don't blame him. Anxiety is hard to understand. So far in this book, we have done a good job of defining a panic attack as *undefinable.* They are impossible to understand for someone who has never had an "attack." While he dealt with his own mental-health struggles, anxiety was not one of them.

Losing my father has been one of the hardest things I've ever faced, and it took a toll on my anxiety.

I never realized that Christmas would be the last time I would ever see or speak to my dad. Christmas 2017, a seemingly ordinary day, turned out to be one of the most significant dates of my life. I replay those final moments with my father repeatedly in my mind.

Even though he couldn't stay long that Christmas, each time I dream about that day, the moments I spent with him become longer and longer. It's as if the dream stretches the time we had together. It was both more than enough time and not enough time at all.

Just months before his passing, I had started a new job, my first "Big Boy" job behind a desk. All I wanted was to share my excitement with him. Shortly after losing him, I got engaged, and I yearned to call him and share the news. Suddenly, the man I hadn't spoken to in two months became the only person I wanted to confide in. Every time I would look at my phone to call him and realize I couldn't, I would feel the familiar quickening of my heart rate at the start of a panic attack.

The combination of a new job, the loss of my father, and my engagement stirred up a whirlwind of emotions within me.

Work became increasingly difficult. I would try to compensate by forcing smiles and laughter, but I started falling behind. Each day, I counted down the minutes until five o'clock, and when I came home, I would drink myself to sleep, only to repeat the same routine the next day.

As you can imagine, this took an enormous toll on my mental health. Panic attacks became a daily occurrence. Some were severe enough to land me in the hospital, mistaken for other symptoms.

I lost interest in the activities that used to bring me joy. Before losing my father, I was a fine-art painter. One of the last paintings I completed was just a week before his passing. But instead of continuing with my art, I sought solace in parties, binge-watching anime, and playing video games until my eyes dried out.

Every night, as I drifted to sleep, I dreamed of spending time with him again. Those dreams felt so incredibly real, and they were filled with the happiest moments of my life at the time.

Yet, no matter how joyful those dreams were, they always ended with a jolt of terror and anxiety. I would wake up feeling a sense of dread and sadness, knowing that he was gone and would never return. All those cherished moments would never be the same.

And that anxiety that started my day would carry and build until it came time to do it all again.

I tried various therapeutic activities. I would journal, occasionally post on his Facebook wall to say hello, and learn to appreciate and cherish the dreams rather than fear them. I focused on the positive memories rather than dwelling on the fact that there would be no more.

However, my psyche was deeply shaken, and the anxiety attacks persisted, growing increasingly intense. I realized I needed to take more drastic measures to halt my mental health decline.

The moral of this story is not simply about the prescriptions and therapies that eventually helped me overcome that dark episode. The true moral of this story is - even in the face of tremendous hardships, **it is possible to climb out of the deepest abyss.** Even when it feels like it can never get better – it will.

Now, five years after losing my father, I can focus on the memories I hold dear. When I think of my dad, I remember him teaching me tennis, taking me out for pizza, or the time he proudly watched me ride my unicycle around the block for the first time. I recall when he brought me and my friends to the mall and gave me twenty dollars of spending money each time—a substantial portion of his wealth just so we could have fun.

I choose to remember the happy times, and with each passing day, I find myself dreading his absence less and less. Now, rather than drink myself to sleep to avoid thinking of him, I instead enjoy his favorite beer, an ice-cold Natty Ice (I know, disgusting) on every Father's Day, birthday, and anniversary of his loss.

Also, in accepting his loss, the anxiety surrounding it has begun to subside. The worst things in life are never an end all, be all.

So, here's to you, Daddio. I pour out a Natty in your honor.

"You don't have to be positive all the time. It's okay to feel sad, angry, annoyed, frustrated, scared, or anxious. Having feelings doesn't make you a negative person. It makes you human."

Lori Deschene

12
A Q&A With My Mom, Linda

L inda, my incredible mother, is an absolute saint. She's not a saint in the traditional sense, but she is the greatest, sweetest, most badass mom a person (especially with anxiety) could ask for. While this book is mostly about my perspective, I also wanted to bring in her unique take on things and allow you to see my story from another perspective.

So, without any more delay, get ready for a special treat—a Q&A session with the one and only Linda. Buckle up and enjoy this delightful detour.

John: Linda, Linda, Linda. The all-famous-coolest mom ever, Linda. In this book, I've talked a lot about how you've helped me immensely throughout my life, and I wanted to ask you a few questions. Do you have a couple of minutes for me?

Linda: Always!

John: Awesome! First, I must address your undeniable popularity. Not only in my friend group but even throughout my entire graduating class of my high school, everyone knew

who "Linda" was. So, I have to ask, how did you become so cool?

Linda: Well, you might be my biggest or really, only fan, but I think my "cool" status is mostly thanks to your perception of me. You see me as cool, and others follow suit.

Although I must admit, I *do* have moments of being pretty cool.

John: Okay, okay, that's enough about you. Let's shift gears and talk about my favorite subject—me. I want to delve into my anxiety throughout the years. So, let's start at the beginning. How did you first notice or become aware of my anxiety, and what were your initial thoughts and feelings?

Linda: Your anxiety symptoms actually began when you were just a toddler. You would frequently complain about stomachaches and had no appetite. You even started losing weight at a young age, which retally concerned me. Initially, I didn't consider mental illness as a possible cause, so I took you to various medical doctors, mainly a gastroenterologist.

At age five, after trying medications to alleviate reflux without success, the doctor performed an endoscopy.

Following the surgery, a tube was inserted through your nose into your stomach, which recorded your activities for forty-eight hours straight. After analyzing the recordings, it became clear that your reflux symptoms diminished significantly during deep sleep, leading them to realize that your condition was not purely medical in nature.

I remember feeling so worried and confused during that time and would often search for answers to understand what you were going through.

John: I remember those tubes. I actually thought they were pretty cool at the time.

When I was *really* young, anxiety attacks were absolutely terrifying for me. I've mentioned before how you were one of the few people who truly understood. How did you manage to calm me down before I started taking medication? And, more importantly, do you have some kind of magical powers?

Linda: If I had magical powers, I would have spared you from going through any of that in the first place!

When the panic attacks began, I didn't immediately recognize them for what they were. Initially, I just thought you were feeling nauseous and might need to vomit.

My main focus was to keep you calm while you were in the midst of an attack, mainly because your dad was trying to sleep for an early day of work and the screaming didn't help.

During those moments, I did my best to soothe you while also trying to understand what you were going through. As a person of strong Christian faith, I also spent a lot of time praying for the ordeal to end.

Many of those nights felt never-ending, lasting for hours on end.

John: There must have been a moment when things started to make sense for you, a realization of what I was going through, especially considering you also experienced anxiety yourself (thanks for the genetics, by the way). Do you think your personal experience with anxiety helped you in supporting me?

Linda: Absolutely, I started having panic attacks when I hit puberty, and they continued for about ten years.

There wasn't a widely known term for my feelings during those early years. My parents thought I was either crazy or using drugs, so I had to hide my struggles from them. I also had to conceal my panic attacks while I was at school.

Since I didn't even know it was a panic attack, the overwhelming thoughts I had were truly confusing. I can vividly recall being terrified that I might do something that would ruin my reputation. There were moments when I sat in class with my mind racing, scared that I would jump on the desk and start screaming, or strip off my clothes and run down the hallway, wondering how far this uncontrollable fear would take me. While you have always feared vomiting during panic attacks, my fear centered around humiliation.

When I entered menopause, my panic attacks resurfaced. This time, I recognized them for what they were since I better understood panic attacks. Fortunately, I knew there were medications available to alleviate them. I sought treatment right away and have been panic-free ever since.

John: That is so important to discuss; the stigma around medication for mental illness needs to be addressed. Our own experiences show that medication can be a lifesaver.

Now, I can only imagine how emotionally and physically draining it must have been to care for a panicking child in public spaces, hoping no one would misconstrue the situation and involve child protective services. Additionally, being there for me every night while I leaned over the toilet must have taken a toll on you. How did you care for yourself amidst pouring so much energy into caring for me?

Linda: Being a Mama Bear has always been ingrained in me. That doesn't mean I didn't have my own moments of breakdowns. Sometimes I would break down, cry, or even raise my voice out of frustration. But most of the time, my focus was on easing your suffering and doing everything I could to make it easier for you.

To recharge myself, I would occasionally retreat to the bathroom. I'd fill the tub with a hot, soothing bubble bath, turn on the fan for some calming white noise, and sometimes even indulge in a glass of wine. It was my little sanctuary where I could briefly escape the stress and reemerge ready to face the challenges of being a mom again.

(Of course, you would usually be sitting on the floor outside the bathroom the whole time, waiting for me to help you again.)

John: I can only imagine how challenging and overwhelming those moments must have been for you, feeling like you were stuck in a real-life crash course of Anxiety Parenting 101. Were there any specific situations or moments where you felt unsure how to support me best?

Linda: Oh, absolutely.

There were instances when we were in the car, and you would suddenly have a panic attack, feeling carsick and terrified of throwing up. You would insist that I pull over so you could escape. Being the accommodating mom that I was, I would calmly find a safe spot to stop, and you would get out and start pacing. During the first few minutes, I could remain calm, and sometimes even for the next few minutes, but if I was in a hurry or exhausted, my patience would wear thin.

The calm and gentle coaxing would transform into a more agitated and louder tone. I remember a couple of occasions when I shouted, "Just get in the car!" much louder than necessary out of frustration and fatigue. It wasn't my proudest moment, but I'm only human.

There were also years when you had teachers who didn't believe that you were struggling with anxiety because you appeared extroverted and relaxed when you weren't experiencing attacks. Dealing with their disbelief and lack of understanding was incredibly frustrating.

Also, when you were younger and medication wasn't considered or the right treatment plan wasn't identified, you began experiencing other physical symptoms that didn't seem directly related to anxiety. It was frightening for me as a mother. Your untreated panic attacks even caused extreme pain, temporary loss of sight, or minor hallucinations, which led doctors to consider other potential conditions like melanoma. Finally, the cause was identified as a Somatic Symptom Disorder from the lengthy extreme stress on your brain, but it was a terrifying experience, and it brought me to tears many times.

Those moments were incredibly challenging, and I had to navigate through them with uncertainty and fear.

John: It amazes me how well you handled what you went through during all of that, and that only helps me appreciate how accommodating you have always been even more so.

After this twenty-eight-year journey of mine, what nuggets of wisdom would you give other parents who are raising an anxiety-ridden child?

Linda:

1. Stay calm as a parent, as your own calmness can help your child calm down more quickly.

2. Always validate your child's feelings, no matter how unusual or irrational they may seem.

3. Understand that there is no one-size-fits-all experience of a panic attack. The feelings, fears, and symptoms can vary for each individual.

4. Recognize that panic attacks are not rational, and it's important to accept and support your child through their emotions and fears.

5. Consider seeking medical advice from experienced doctors who have dealt with a range of symptoms associated with anxiety.

6. Lastly, get a pedicure on weekends. You deserve it!

These tips encompass the importance of empathy, patience, understanding, and self-care in navigating the journey of raising a child with anxiety.

John: I was *incredibly* lucky to have someone like you (and some of those old wise doctors) in my life, but obviously, not everyone gets that lucky and has to bury their anxiety. And unfortunately, you can't be a mom to all those people. What would you say to all of them if you could?

Linda: It's going to be okay. It will *always* be okay.

Take a moment to relax your body, starting from your shoulders down to your fingertips and toes, one body part at a time.

And most importantly, don't forget to breathe.

John: I see what you did there.

Next question, did my anxiety ever make you want to pull your hair out or scream into a pillow? How did you manage to keep your cool and not join me in the circus of anxiety? Amid all the chaos, there must have been some standout moments that left a lasting impression. Share with us one of those memories from the anxiety rollercoaster ride we've been on together.

Linda: Oh, I know what story you are referring to.

I definitely had moments when your anxiety felt overwhelming, and I wanted to pull my hair out or scream into a pillow. It was a challenging journey, but I realized that losing my cool wouldn't help either of us. I had to find ways to keep calm amid the chaos, often taking deep breaths and reminding myself to stay patient and understanding.

However, there was one incident when you were around twelve or thirteen and experiencing an intense panic attack. At that difficult moment, I made the decision to tell you that you couldn't sleep in my room. I admit: I had a meltdown and ended up yelling at you repeatedly. It was a regrettable reaction on my part, and you ended up sleeping on the floor in the hallway that night.

Looking back, I realize that none of us are perfect, and we all have our breaking points. But what matters is how we learn and grow from those experiences. I've learned from that meltdown and consciously tried to handle difficult situations with more patience and understanding.

John: Panic attacks can be just as hard for the caretakers as they are for the freak-outers.

Okay, so far in this book, I have liked to have fun and laugh at some of the more fun times looking back, and our conversation has been pretty serious. Any funny anxiety stories you'd like to share?

Linda: Remember the time I had to drop everything and drive up to you in Boston because you were in the middle of a four-hour panic attack?

Remember how you forgot to take your meds, which threw you into a week's worth of panic attacks?

I remember.

During one of your "panic attack walks," on that trip I jokingly said to you, "If you ever forget to take your medications again, I'll beat the shit out of you." Now, let's clarify that this is our unique sense of humor and is by no means abusive. But in response, while your teeth were chattering and you were shaking, you looked at me and said, "*Mom... now is not the time!*"

We still laugh about that moment to this day. It's one of those lighthearted memories that brings some comic relief amidst the challenges we've faced together.

John: I could totally take you in a fight. However, everyone knows we are best friends, so do we owe any thanks to my illness?

Linda: You know, I never really considered it, but now that you mention it, perhaps we do owe some thanks to your illness. Going through those challenging times together has forged a unique bond between us.

John: Okay, final question. Pineapple on Pizza, yes, or no?

Linda: *No.*

"Don't let happy days just pass you by."

Closure in Moscow, "Happy Days"

DEEP BREATHS | 109

13
Relationships Are Hard Enough, Damnit.

You read the title—relationships are tough. Well, not all relationships, of course. Some relationships just click, like finding the perfect pair of socks in a messy drawer. Those are the people who become your ride-or-die crew from the get-go.

Like, that one person who noticed you missed your first few days of school (from anxiety) and wanted to check-in. Or maybe it was as simple as someone who introduced themselves with a casual, "Wanna be friends?" and has been by your side for over two decades. Sometimes it's easy, but most relationships don't just fall into your lap.

When it comes to friendships, making a true friend often means peeling back the layers, letting your guard down, and revealing those parts of yourself you don't show to just anyone. It's about trust. And while gaining someone's trust may not be the hardest part, trusting others is where many of us stumble.

Especially those of us with anxiety.

Anxiety comes in various shapes and sizes, and we've talked a lot about mine. But let's take a minute to discuss others, namely those with social anxiety, a form of anxiety that most people can relate to on some level. I mean we have all stood in front of a large crowd, ready to give a speech with our palms as sweaty as

Eminem's. Sure, that can induce some anxiety in anyone. But for those with social anxiety? They might as well have forgotten what sleep feels like for the past week, thanks to the all-consuming dread of waiting to give this presentation.

People with social anxiety often struggle to open up about themselves. They might avoid eating in public just to dodge the nerve-racking experience of ordering from a server. And dating? It's a whole new level of opening up.

Social anxiety can be a significant roadblock on the path to a healthy relationship, but truly any form of anxiety can hijack your chances at a positive and productive dating experience.

And it doesn't even start on the first date. No, the butterflies in your stomach begin at the very first interaction. Let's set the scene in the digital realm, since we're well into the twenty-first century.

You receive the first message. Do you reply immediately? Will that make you appear too eager? Maybe you should wait a bit, play it cool. But if you wait too long, they might think you don't care. It's a constant battle between response timing and perception.

Oh boy, it's a rollercoaster. Trust me, I've been on that ride more times than I care to admit. But hey, everyone says, "Just be yourself, and everything will work out." So, you muster the courage to respond authentically, but then they don't reply fast enough.

Doubts creep in. What if your answer wasn't good enough? What if they suddenly decided you were the ugliest creature to roam the earth in the two minutes since you answered, and now they want nothing to do with you?

The "what if" game, the root of most anxiety, eats away at you. And it doesn't stop there. The first date, oh, the first date. It's a challenge in itself, but the panic attack that tempts you to cancel the date is even harder to handle.

If I may, let me share a personal experience.

Once upon a time, I landed a date – a first date - with an exceptionally, *exceptionally*, handsome man, but I couldn't help but wonder, *Why in the world would they be interested in me?*

We scheduled the date, carefully selecting a public space for both safety and anxiety purposes. Two weeks to prepare seemed like plenty of time. But, with that amount of time, the dread began to build. Seven days left. Six days left. Five days left. Should I reschedule? Maybe I need more time. No, no, I can handle this. Four days left... Never mind, let's cancel.

I could go on with this story, but the truth is, this isn't just one isolated incident. I didn't embark on a fairytale romance and find "my person" in a heartbeat. No, I've dated and dated and dated some more, battling anxiety along the way.

The hardest part about dating with anxiety wasn't always the feelings I experienced; sometimes, it was the impact those feelings had on the other person. From canceling plans to abruptly leaving in the middle of said dates, anxiety has caused its fair share of disruptions in my relationship life. And the unfortunate reality is that not everyone understands. Nobody enjoys canceled plans, but when you cancel plans because you're "anxious" with someone who has never experienced a panic attack, forgiveness isn't always guaranteed, especially if it becomes a pattern.

I have found that it has been vital to surround myself with people who truly understand me. My closest friendships have always been rooted in a deep understanding and unwavering compassion when it comes to my panic disorder. Having someone who truly comprehends my struggles allows me to open up and express myself as I should—to let the true colors of my wild and crazy personality shine through without worry of what people are thinking of me, for better or worse.

So, as we conclude this short chapter, remember this: whether it's a job interview, a presentation, or a first date, *you've got this*. There's a good chance that someone else in the room, or even sitting across from you, feels the same way. And if all else fails, just picture everyone else in their underwear. That's what they say, right?

And finally - to *my* best friends and partners who have always understood: Thank you.

"The only person who can pull me down is myself,
and I'm not going to let myself pull me down anymore."

C. JoyBell C.

14
Unexpected Allies

S uppose you suffer from anxiety or panic attacks. In that case, you may have been in a similar situation once or twice to what I am about to recount. Or rather, you may be the person or type of person I am about to reference, and if so, I would like to thank you in advance.

Many people need help understanding us or what we go through. However, occasionally someone comes around who acts as the weighted blanket you need in a moment of panic. They don't just immediately understand *you*, but they understand exactly what you are going through. They are there for you in a sea of people who are not.

These people are our firefighters in a crisis. They rush into our burning building of a panic attack with no preparation and no equipment. They are not necessarily just there to put out our fire, they are there to save us and get us out of the fire altogether.

I would like to share three stories of people who have saved me from my very own fires.

*　　　*　　　*

It was a wedding, and naturally, I indulged in a bit too much drinking. To make things worse, the bartender happened to be a close friend of the bride, a guy from a small town who had quite the talent for pouring heavy-handed drinks. And, in my defense, I went to that wedding with one goal in mind: to have an epic, unforgettable time.

The night was mostly good. We danced, took photos. Everything was going great.

Until it wasn't. And for that, we owe thanks to none other than cotton candy vodka shots.

Everyone seemed to be ordering them. You would think it was the cotton candy vodka apocalypse, and this was the last of the supply. So naturally, I also thought the same and enjoyed one or five too many of these sugary death traps.

Soon the night seemed like a blur of dancing and laughter. Judging by the pictures, my partner and I had the time of our lives—I just wish I could remember more of it. Regardless, it was going great.

But then, that fateful and fearful moment arrived, and I saw it in my partner's eyes—the shot that pushed the limits of his tolerance and threatened my biggest fear.

In a panic, we ran outside to the parking lot. And wouldn't you know it, my worst nightmare happened right before my very eyes—he threw up everywhere.

And, to clarify, this happened *during* my impressive streak of thirteen years without witnessing, smelling, or being anywhere near vomit. Seeing my partner in that state triggered a primal response deep within me.

While my partner was busy purging his woes, my body decided that it wanted to join in on the fun. But instead of letting loose the contents of my stomach, I found myself pacing back and forth, stealing glances at my partner, dry-heaving, and caught in the throes of a full-blown panic attack.

I was a teary mess, alone in a nearly empty parking lot while everyone comforted my projectile-vomiting partner.

And then, like a guardian angel, a close friend of mine appeared by my side, offering support to me. Me, the one who was crying about someone else throwing up, not even the one getting sick myself.

"No, no, help him. I'm fine," I begged, desperate for her to redirect her attention. But she saw through my protests. She understood that at that moment, what I needed most was someone by my side, reminding me that I wasn't alone in this storm of emotions.

With her support, and many others, we managed to make it home safely. My mom, always ready to come to the rescue, came to pick us up.

She may have encountered a few overzealous partygoers trying to hit on her along the way, and the soundtrack of the ride home consisted mainly of both mine and my partner's tearful cries, but hey, at least we made it home in one piece.

Life has its unexpected twists and turns, and sometimes all it takes is a friend who sees beyond your protests and sticks by your side when you need them the most. So, here's to those unlikely heroes who show up in parking lots, wipe away our tears, and help us navigate the messiness of life, one unpredictable wedding at a time.

*   *   *

My family is riddled with mental illness. We are like trading card collectors, or Pokémon Trainers trying to catch 'em all. My mom, as you know, had her hands full trying to navigate life with a mentally ill son, and often relied on her sisters for support.

Caring for a child like me was no easy task, but finding someone who understood enough to help, was even harder. It takes finding someone with an understanding of anxiety disorders to care for or watch over a screaming child during a panic attack.

Cue my other mentally ill aunts.

Sometimes, in the realm of mental health, the best support comes from those who fight similar battles. It's like a secret club, and maybe that's why you picked up this book—to find solace in the shared experiences of kindred spirits, to join the club.

Luckily for me, I had my fair share of like-minded people surrounding me, ready to pull me from the safety net I had made of my mom.

My aunts became my pillars of strength, my refuge when I needed a break from the world. They would swoop in and offer a break to my mom, granting her a well-deserved mental retreat from time to time.

For me, that meant stepping into their world, which was both terrifying and exhilarating. Leaving my mom's side at such a young age felt like a death sentence. I couldn't let go of one safe space without frantically seeking another.

One of my aunts was an anxiety whisperer, a master of distraction. Spending weekends with her was like entering a secret sanctuary of understanding. She just got it, you know? And when panic threatened to consume me whole, she'd pull out her bag of tricks, diverting my attention with games, adventures, and *plenty* of laughter.

Then there was my other aunt—let's call her the Queen of Disorders. She had a list of mental disorders longer than a CVS receipt. Though she didn't often babysit me, we did have plenty of late-night sessions, deep-diving into the intricacies of our individual battles. We'd compare notes—trade cards— exchanging badges of honor from our personal wars against mental illness. "Oh, you feel that way too? Welcome to the club!" became a frequent reminder we would share that meant we weren't alone in this crazy and chaotic life.

I'll never forget one particular night when we stayed up late at night as we deep dove into our minds. It was like a support group meeting, except with more snacks and a hammock mishap.

We found solace in each other's stories, weaving a blanket of understanding and resilience. I never thought that anyone would understand me the way she had.

Now, whether biological or chosen, I understand that not everyone has the luxury of a supportive family. Loneliness can be an unwelcome friend on this journey called an anxious life. But speaking from experience, I implore you to seek those who understand you. Maybe that means joining online discussions. Maybe you find a professional, who will understand you on a whole new level. Perhaps it just means revisiting this book multiple times—I will always be here.

Remember, even in the darkest storms, there's always a glimmer of light waiting to guide you through the storm. And sometimes, that light comes from unexpected allies who understand your battles because they've fought similar ones themselves. Together, we can navigate this storm of mental health, finding strength in unity and embracing humor in the absurdity of it all.

*   *   *

Middle school was an incredibly challenging time for me. As I mentioned before, I coped with my anxiety by being loud and acting out—compensating. This meant that I never let my walls down to allow anyone to see the real me or understand what I was truly going through. Well, except for one person—my middle-school nurse.

When starting a new school with my long list of disorders, it always meant meeting with the staff and having some difficult conversations.

"Hey, I'm medicated, so I may fall asleep during class."

"Hey, I'm on restricted medication, you might need to lock it in a secure box for when I need it."

"Hey, if I cry and scream for no reason, you may need to break that box open and throw this medication down my throat."

These discussions became a regular occurrence whenever I moved to a new school district, which happened quite frequently actually.

For most of the new staff, these meetings were just a standard part of their job. They would encounter a new student with a disability (which for me, they often considered minor) and sit through a meeting they probably didn't want to attend, listening to all the details. And I don't blame them—meetings suck.

But, for my middle-school nurse, this particular meeting meant something more.

My middle-school nurse became one of the most important people in my life during one of the toughest periods of my life I've faced. While I compensated for my anxiety by acting out, she saw right through it. She saw me for who I truly was and didn't pay attention to the bratty middle schooler I pretended to be.

Throughout those middle-school years, my panic attacks reached an all-time high in intensity. Maybe it was puberty, but I doubt it as I was a late, late bloomer.

When my panic attacks would hit me during school, I couldn't shake or cry in the middle of class. I couldn't just get up and run out of class or I would make a fool of myself.

I had nowhere to go, except my one safe space—the nurse's office. Whenever I went to the nurse with a panic attack, her approach was always the same: understanding and distraction. First, we would talk through what I was feeling, and she would bring me down to earth and make me feel *normal*. Then, we would play games to distract me to the other side. We would solve complicated math problems together on her computer or play speech games back and forth—whatever it took to divert my attention from my gripping panic attack, and stop my seizure like shaking.

To this day, I'm not entirely sure why she was as exceptional as she was. Maybe she had dealt with similar issues herself or maybe she was a caretaker for someone else like me. Whatever the reason, there's only one thing that truly matters to me:

To my middle-school nurse, I want to express my heartfelt gratitude to you for being my guiding light during the storm.

Your unwavering support and understanding made a world of difference in my life, and I will always cherish the moments we spent together. Thank you for seeing beyond my anxiety-driven facade and for being a beacon of comfort when I needed it the most. You made an impact that will stay with me forever.

And to all the nurses who help kids like me, continue being our firefighters. You are a hero more than you know.

Even when you won't send us home for a fake bellyache.

"You are not alone in this. You are loved and supported, even on the darkest days."

Unknown

15
A Showdown with Yourself

Imagine yourself on a camping adventure, deep in the heart of nature, when suddenly, in the dead of night, a pressing need to relieve yourself strikes. Ah, the joys of nature's call! But the campsite's bathroom is a considerable distance away, and halfway there, your biggest fear comes true: an enormous bear lurks in the shadows, ready to pounce and block your path to the latrine. Now, what do you do in such a nerve-wracking scenario? Do you succumb to fear, allowing it to paralyze you? No way! You summon the spirit of a bold explorer, muster your courage, and look that bear right in the eye, defiantly declaring, "Not today, bear! I am determined to reach the bathroom, and you won't stand in my way!" Maybe you even punch that bear right in the furry face.

All right, let's set the record straight: that was an analogy. No actual bears were harmed or encountered in the making of this scenario. As you may have guessed, I'm referring to anxiety—a common theme in this book. But the underlying message remains the same: sometimes, we must summon our inner strength, look our anxiety right in the eyes and say, "Not today!"

Admittedly, mastering this skill was not a walk in the park for me, and I'm hardly a master. When anxiety strikes, it's all too tempting to give up, allowing our bodies to shake, our minds to race, and our thoughts to spiral into chaos. Putting a halt to these instinctual responses requires quite a bit of effort—it's like those "try not to laugh" challenges that somehow end up making you laugh even harder.

Confronting anxiety takes more than just sheer willpower. It demands courage—an unwavering determination to face the storm head-on. When that foreboding black cloud of anxiety rolls in, obscuring our vision and distorting our perception of reality, it becomes easy to lose our sense of direction. We find ourselves begging to escape, yet the smog of anxiety blinds us and leaves us disoriented. Which way should we turn? How do we find our way out?

But, facing anxiety doesn't involve escaping the smog entirely; instead, it entails convincing ourselves that the smog is not real— that we can see clearly, and that there's truly nothing to fear. It is seeing through the illusionary mind trick.

And let's be honest—that is a far from an easy feat.

Lately, I've been honing my skills in dispelling that suffocating smog of anxiety. I've trained my brain to respond with thoughts such as, "You've never thrown up before, so why would it suddenly happen now?" or "Sure, you might feel the urge to flee this plane, but let's be rational here—there's no immediate danger (or parachutes)." These cognitive exercises have become my trusted allies, skilled at dispersing the dark clouds of anxiety that threaten to engulf me.

I'm my experiences, I have found that the key to making these thoughts effective lies in catching the anxiety storm early, intercepting the thoughts before they gain momentum. There becomes a point during a full-blown panic attack where these rationalizations become entirely ineffective. That's why it's crucial to nip it in the bud—to rise to your feet, take charge of the situation, and stop the anxiety train dead in its tracks before it picks up an unstoppable speed.

And again—it is not easy. Imagine finding yourself at the mercy of a robber, staring down the barrel of a gun, and instead of quivering with fear, you meet your assailant's gaze with an audacious smile, confidently asserting, "You won't harm me today, because I won't allow it!" That's the level of unwavering rationality required to tell your own anxiety a resounding "no." But believe it or not, when it comes to anxiety, such an approach can disarm it entirely.

Recently I did just this. I was in a meeting—my favorite place— and just the thought of being there began to set my mind and heart racing. The idea of being trapped in this meeting with nowhere to go was the catalyst. What if I get sick? What if I need to run? What if, what if, what if?

But I couldn't let it happen. It took looking myself right in the eyes (metaphorically) and saying, "You are fine. There is nothing to be scared of, and even if the worst happens, you just leave the meeting. You got this." And it worked. I calmed myself down before it got out of hand.

So, I implore you to take charge the next time you sense those relentless what-if scenarios piling up or feel the suffocating smog of anxiety enveloping your senses. Clear the air, muster your inner strength, and look yourself in the mirror, resolutely declaring, "No." Stop that train of worry dead in its tracks. Remember, you possess an innate power within you to overcome these anxiety-fueled battles, one defiant "not today" at a time.

You've got this too.

"There is hope, even when your brain
tells you there isn't."

John Green

16
It's Not Fair

Whatever your relationship with anxiety is, we can all agree on one thing: it is not fair. Nope, not fair at all. It's like anxiety has a twisted sense of humor, playing tricks on us when we least expect it. But hey, life isn't always fair, right?

Imagine it is the night before your first dance recital. Excitement and nerves intertwine like awkwardly synchronized dance partners. But what's that? Anxiety decides to take it too far and crash the party with a bit of flair. You end up with anxiety poops, a delightful little surprise right before your grand debut on stage. Talk about unfairness! It's like anxiety has a vendetta against dignity.

And that's just the tip of the unfairness iceberg. Living each day in fear, dreading what the next moment might bring, is not fair. Relying on medication to keep those irrational fears in check? Definitely not fair. Missing the SpongeBob Squarepants movie? Not Fair.

Missing out on lunch dates with friends because anxiety decides to rain on your parade? Unfair. And when your friends use anxiety as an excuse to bail on lunch? Yeah, that's unfair too.

And it is certainly not fair watching someone you love struggle with anxiety.

We've all been there, caught up in those thoughts of "Why me?" It's like we're playing a game of existential bingo, and anxiety is our free square. We wonder why we were chosen to be the anxiety sufferers out of all the people on this spinning ball we call Earth. Well, I'll tell you what's not fair: that train of thought. It's time to kick it to the curb and embrace a new perspective.

In the wise words of Lady Gaga, "Baby, you were born this way."

Yes, you, my friend, deserve to love yourself for all your strengths and despite all your weaknesses. It took me a while to learn that lesson, but boy, am I glad I did. You see, I've always had confidence in myself, but for the longest time, there was one thing I despised about myself: my panic attacks. I hated myself for missing school, for not being able to do what other kids did, and for needing my mom as a chaperone in life. I hated myself for struggling when other people just got to be normal. I hated myself, and it was not fair.

But if I could turn back time and have a little chat with my past self, I'd say this: Life isn't fair, kiddo. We all have our struggles. When we struggle so badly, we look at everyone around us and put on blinders to their struggles. It becomes so easy to feel sorry for yourself, you forget to feel sorry for others.

While I was busy wallowing in my own pain, I failed to see the battles others were fighting. There was a classmate growing up with only one parent after losing the other, a new kid struggling to make friends due to language barriers, and even family members dealing with their own mental-health issues. Even my dad had his own daily struggles, which I didn't acknowledge.

But here's the thing—acknowledging the pain of others helps us realize that we're not alone. It's like joining a support group where everyone's got their own set of quirks and baggage—that secret society. I began to see my pain as a tool rather than a handicap. By sharing my experiences, I could lend a helping hand to others who were also navigating the treacherous waters of anxiety.

And so, I did just that. People started gravitating toward me, pouring their hearts out within minutes of meeting me. It's like I have a beacon of compassion and understanding above my head.

If that's the case, then I owe a big thank you to my anxiety.

Maybe, just maybe, it *is* fair that I've gone through what I have.

Distraction is the best Medicine

I have found that distraction is often the best medicine when it comes to panic attacks. So, here are thirty-five unconventional ways you can distract yourself the next time you feel anxious:

1. Dance. I don't care where you are—just dance.
2. Knit a sweater
3. Find paper *fast* and do the first origami pattern you remember.
4. Do some Sudoku.
5. Find that project you started a few months ago, and begin it again.
6. Play the nearest item to you as if it were a musical instrument.
7. Find the nearest book, turn to a random page, and read a random paragraph.
8. Begin a vision board.
9. Take a picture of the first person you see.
10. Cook some food!
11. Take a walk.
12. Close your eyes, and pick a show on Netflix.
13. Play a board game with a friend—or yourself.
14. Check-in on the Duolingo Owl you have been ignoring.
15. Start a puzzle.

16. Pretend it is Thanksgiving, and list everything you are thankful for in your life. Out loud or in your head—your choice.

17. Write two five-digit numbers and try to multiply them.

18. Run.

19. Take a shower and draw pictures on the wall with soap.

20. Drink some tea.

21. Host a tea party with some stuffed animals.

22. Clean out that overflowing closet you have been ignoring.

23. Play mini golf with items near you.

24. Invent a board game.

25. Learn to solve a Rubik's Cube.

26. Now do it with your feet.

27. Create a stop-motion film with items around your house.

28. Turn your driveway into a work of art with sidewalk chalk.

29. Sing at the top of your lungs.

30. Juggle the three nearest items.

31. Count the hairs on your arm.

32. Come up with a secret handshake with your imaginary friend.

33. Write a book.

17
Ghosts of Panic Past

Brains are stupid.

Seriously, why do they have to take something as simple as a fleeting thought and turn it into a full-blown panic attack? It's like our own brains have a twisted sense of humor, playing tricks on us just when we least expect it. But hey, I guess that's why I'm here, talking about my anxiety. So, let's dive into this present moment, where my brain is *currently* playing its favorite game of panic-attack roulette.

Currently, while writing this chapter, I am having a major panic attack.

I'm sitting here, fingers trembling like a salsa dancer on caffeine, trying to type out this chapter while my brain is doing somersaults. It's a sight to behold, let me tell you. If only you could see the words on this page right now, not a single word typed correctly. *Editing this is going to be a wild ride, but I digress.*

Let's talk about what triggered this little episode. Lately, my anxiety has been back in full swing. It's like anxiety thought, *hey, I've been on hiatus for a while, let's make a grand entrance and wreak havoc in our favorite anxious person's life.*

Thanks, anxiety, you always know how to throw a party.

We all know by now that I am terrified of throwing up, and the attack today—and all attacks recently—are no different. That fear over the past few months has spiraled and evolved into so many more attacks, which currently have a hold on me. I'm scared of car rides because what if I get motion sickness and puke all over the upholstery? Mornings have become the ultimate suspense thriller, where waking up with a slight touch of nausea feels like the opening scene of a horror movie. And forget about eating. Each bite – every single one – I have to choke down as I convince myself it is okay to eat, that I won't get sick for no reason. Every bite eaten is a victory.

A few mornings ago, I faced a panic attack so severe, it ended up lasting nearly all day long. I woke up nauseous and the panic took over. I was four hours away from home visiting my family and friends back in New Jersey, which meant I was not in my safe space. With the increase of my heart rate and the spiraling of my thoughts, a tinge of nausea turned into what felt I had drunk a gallon of spoiled milk. Thank goodness for anti-nausea medication, right? Wrong. Turns out, the nausea wasn't a result of some wicked stomach bug, or expired milk. It was my anxiety itself, my fear of being nauseous causing the nausea and no amount of treating the nausea itself would help.

In retrospect, it's clear that I was treating the wrong symptom. Silly me, thinking anti-nausea meds could quiet the storm of anxiety brewing inside. But at that moment, all I could think was, *I'm going to puke, and nothing can save me!*

Dramatic, I know, but panic attacks have a way of turning even the smallest hiccup into a full-blown volcanic eruption.

But guess what? I made it through that day. Sure, my food intake only consisted of a sad smoothie from White Castle and a few pretzels, but I survived unscathed.

Or so I thought.

Back to today. Just this morning, I was having a fabulous time watching *RuPaul's Drag Race*. I am in the midst of a total rewatch, and today's episode was the grand finale of season seven. But as I enjoyed the climactic episode, out of nowhere, my brain decided to bring up that memory from New Jersey and go, *hey, remember when you felt like you rode the world's worst rollercoaster for twenty-four hours straight? Let's do that again!*

And just like that, my mind was hijacked. Sasha Velour's epic reveal on the television took a backseat to my spiraling thoughts. *What if this attack lasts forever? What if it's even worse than last time? What if—horror of horrors—I actually do throw up?* The what-ifs danced around in my mind, mocking me.

And now, here I am, still caught in the whirlwind of my thoughts, wondering when this anxiety tornado will finally calm down. I sit here, sipping chamomile tea like it's the elixir of serenity and clutching an isopropyl alcohol wipe and trying to sniff the nausea away. I sit here, knowing that I need to treat the anxiety first and the nausea will go away. I sit here waiting for the Xanax to kick in and convince my brain of that, which I know to be true. I sit here haunted by past attacks- attacks from weeks ago breeding new fears today.

I sit here, haunted by my own ghosts of panic past.

"Your mental health journey is unique to you. Don't compare it to others. Progress is progress, no matter how small."

Unknown

18
What Comes Next?

Throughout the pages of this book, we have delved into the intricacies of my past, exploring the depths of my experiences. In the previous chapter, we even embarked on a journey through the present, grounding ourselves in the reality of the moment. But now, a question lingers: What lies ahead for me?

The truth is, I don't know. The future remains uncertain. How do I prepare for the unpredictable nature of what lies beyond the horizon? How do I equip myself to face the unknown? The answer resides in the wisdom I have gathered from my past battles, the fragments of knowledge I cling to as I venture into uncharted territory.

Reflecting upon moments of unparalleled bliss and triumph, we can gather strength and courage, recognizing that more moments of joy await us in the tapestry of time. Anticipating the good and embracing the bad that life has in store become essential on our journey. And as for the trials and tribulations that may cross our path, we confront them with unwavering determination, undeterred by fear, for we carry the lessons of our past like shields of resilience on our back.

That's right, we are badass knights in this analogy. Let's continue with that.

When contemplating the future, worry serves us no purpose. It merely casts a shadow over our present, obscuring our vision and hindering our progress. Instead, we can place our trust in the journey itself, acknowledging that life has an uncanny way of molding us through hardship. Each challenge we face becomes an opportunity for growth, a testament to our capacity for adaptation and transformation. A sword in our hand.

As for me, I stand resolute in my purpose. Anxiety has been an unwelcome companion throughout my life, an evil dragon in the castle that has threatened to consume me. Yet, it has also been a catalyst for personal transformation. It has ignited a flame of empathy and understanding within me, enabling me to forge deeper connections with my fellow travelers. Is my journey with anxiety over? No, it is an ongoing battle, a dance of resilience and vulnerability. I never defeat the dragon, just subdue him, and await his return. But with each step I take, I emerge stronger and more equipped to face the future head-on, sword and shield in hand.

The path that stretches before me holds both shadows and sunlight. It is a path I am prepared to tread, utilizing the tools and insights I have acquired to navigate its twists and turns. However, my future is not solely centered around my own growth and well-being. It is also about extending a helping hand to others who find themselves navigating their own labyrinthine journeys and fighting their own dragons. Through my struggles and triumphs, I have come to appreciate the universality of adversity. Life, in its vast tapestry, weaves threads of challenge for us all. And if there is one legacy I wish to leave behind, it is utilizing my experiences to uplift and support those who may feel lost or overwhelmed and make it through our adventures. The times I use my sword and shield for good.

Writing this book was born from that very purpose—to offer solace, understanding, and guidance to those who may find themselves wrestling with anxiety. Whether you stumbled upon these words amid a bestseller list or became the only fifth and final reader, if this book helps but one person, I have done my job. If my words can resonate, if they can provide solace or inspiration, then I have fulfilled my mission, as a brave knight, or I suppose bard now, in this journey of life.

So, as I stand on the precipice of the unknown, I will march forward with my head held high, drawing strength from the depths of my being. I will embrace the terrifying uncertainty, knowing that within myself lies the power to confront whatever awaits. And in my triumphs, I will extend a hand to others, creating a ripple effect of compassion and resilience that transcends my individual life.

The future beckons, and it is time for me to step into the beautiful unknown of what awaits.

Gosh, what a beautiful war cry against anxiety.

"Humor is mankind's greatest blessing."

Mark Twain

19
Laughing Through the Tears

As we reach the conclusion of this book, I want to reflect on the journey we have taken together throughout these pages. From the depths of anxiety to the peaks of laughter, we have explored the vast landscape of my own and all human emotion—especially concerning those of us with a panic disorder. From SpongeBob Squarepants to Lady Gaga- from *RuPaul's Drag Race* to nights with my head on the toilet, we have covered a lot of ground.

When I decided to write this book, I was unsure what the message would be. Was it a self-help book? Was it an educational book? A standard memoir? After coming to my final words, I am proud to say it was all of those. It was an all-encompassing manual with plenty of lessons, but the one I would like to leave you with is: Don't take yourself too seriously, laugh, have fun, and don't blame yourself for what you go through.

Throughout these pages, we have explored the complexities of anxiety—just how bad it can get. We have talked about the crazy thoughts *I* have experienced, and I have repeated that panic attacks resoundingly suck. Like Spongebob and Patrick on the quest for Shell City, we have taken a journey throughout my life and all its unexpected turns and hardships.

However, an unexpected turn in the journey of this book for myself was how positively I was able to talk about my anxiety - a shackle around my ankle my entire life, after reflecting, is empowering me to keep moving.

And, like the end of that fateful SpongeBob Squarepants movie, I have discussed how important it is to sometimes just be a Goofy Goober. Find joy in life—even during pain.

Laughter is a best friend, a bubble of joy that rises to the surface when life seems unbearable. It serves as a reminder that amidst the chaos, we can find solace and strength. Remember a time you laughed so hard that tears streamed down your face?

Extreme emotions tend to be the ones that stay in our mind, so rather than focus on the dark side of that, create new positive extreme emotions to carry in the storybook of your life. Don't let the extreme sadness bring you down, instead let the moments of extreme happiness be the ones that you carry with you.

Never forget to laugh at the moments when sometimes you consider jumping out a plane window to get away from an invisible fear.

Those vulnerable and raw experiences that our crazy brain creates reveal what it is to be human. They teach us that life is messy, unpredictable, and sometimes downright uncomfortable.

Yet, even in those moments, I personally have found strength and resilience. In looking back and smiling, I have learned to embrace my imperfections and find the humor and absurdity in it all.

As we navigate our mazes of anxiety, it is crucial to remember that laughter is not just a temporary escape; it is one of many coping mechanisms that empower ourselves to move forward. Rather than letting the ball and chain keep us from moving, smiling and laughing give us the strength to drag that chain behind us and keep pushing forward.

When we can laugh at the pain, we rob anxiety of its power over us. It is like looking the universe in the face and saying, "Try to break me—I will just laugh about it later."

Laughter is also infectious. It spreads like a ripple in the water, influencing all those around us—because believe it or not, our lives are not the only hard ones, and likely *far* from the hardest. Through laughter, and a refusal to take our problems too seriously, we can become beacons of hope, showing others too that in the darkest moments, laughter can be a guiding light.

The truth is: life will always throw us curveballs, and we may not be ready to catch them. In the moments after that curveball breaks our nose, we may struggle to recover, but what I have found so important in life is to look back and think about just how funny you looked with that swollen face.

As I bid farewell to these pages, I begin to realize that maybe this book is not just about anxiety. This book shares stories that allow us to embrace our vulnerabilities, no matter what they may be. This book is about finding strength in the chaos. It is about navigating life's uncertainties, with the confidence of a brave knight, the absurdity of Spongebob and Patrick, and the positivity we all deserve.

Before I leave you, I remind you to carry with you all the tools I have equipped you with. Carry your own adversity toolkit no matter what that may be, with honor. Remember the memories we shared and the laughter that I hope echoed through these pages.

And remember, even if you are laughing through the tears, you are *still smiling.*

"You are so much stronger than you think."

Unknown

20
A Letter to My Past Self

Dear John,

I hope this letter finds you when you need it most.

Maybe it's your first day of school and you are worried that you won't be able to make it through the day. Or, maybe, this letter finds you on one of the many mornings when you are sitting in Linda's car outside the school because you just can't get yourself to go in. Maybe this letter even finds you after four hours of a full-blown panic attack as you drift to sleep on your soccer ball pillow.

Whenever you read this, know that I'm here to offer some nuggets of wisdom to help you navigate the stormy seas of anxiety.

Now, listen up, my anxious friend. It won't be a walk in the park. Each panic attack will make you feel like the world is imploding - like the universe has conspired against your peace of mind. The intensity will grow with each episode, and you'll be convinced that life as you know it is over. But guess what? Thousands of attacks later, I can confidently tell you that life doesn't get stuck in that abyss forever. In fact, you'll spend more time feeling happy than being trapped in panic's clutches. I promise.

Your journey won't be *without* its challenges. Some of the toughest moments will make those anxiety attacks rear their ugly heads with a vengeance. But guess what again? You'll face them head-on and come out on top. You're tougher than you think.

So yes, your life will be full of some really, really hard times. But your life will also be filled with incredible moments. Moments that will make your heart soar, your smile reach ear to ear, and your soul dance with joy. And you know what? Those moments will outweigh the bad ones by a long shot. They're the moments that make life worth living, even amid the stormy weather.

Sure, your panic attacks won't magically disappear, and yes, more hurdles will come. But what truly matters is this: no matter how severe they get or how long they last, you always make it through. Every. Single. Time. Remember that.

You'll emerge from these trials as a stronger, more resilient version of yourself. The lessons you'll learn from this rollercoaster ride called anxiety will shape you into a person overflowing with empathy and compassion. You'll become a guiding light for others navigating their own rocky paths.

Don't let the weight of anxiety anchor you down, preventing you from swimming toward the shore of your dreams.

Work hard through each moment of fear. Fight with every fiber of your being and remind yourself that you can weather this storm.

Equip yourself with a sword and shield for the battle, and remember to laugh, even through tears. Take it one moment at a time, savor the happy moments that come your way, and above all else...

... just breathe.

Mental Health Resources

Mental health is a battle, but is never a battle you have to face alone. Below is a list of resources you can use to seek help in your own battle.

Hotlines and Helplines

National Suicide Prevention Lifeline: 1-800-273-TALK (1-800-273-8255)

Crisis Text Line: Text "HELLO" to 741741

National Alliance on Mental Illness (NAMI) Helpline: 1-800-950-NAMI (1-800-950-6264)

Substance Abuse and Mental Health Services Administration (SAMHSA) National Helpline: 1-800-662-HELP (1-800-662-4357)

Online Support and Information

NAMI (National Alliance on Mental Illness): www.nami.org

Mental Health America (MHA): www.mhanational.org

Anxiety and Depression Association of America (ADAA): www.adaa.org

PsychCentral: www.psychcentral.com

Therapy and Counseling

BetterHelp: www.betterhelp.com
Talkspace: www.talkspace.com

Apps and Tools

Calm: Meditation and sleep app.
Headspace: Guided meditation and mindfulness.
Daylio: Mood tracking and journaling app.
Woebot: AI-driven mental health chatbot.

Books and Reading

"The Anxiety and Phobia Workbook" by Edmund Bourne: A comprehensive guide to managing anxiety.
"The Happiness Project" by Gretchen Rubin: Exploring happiness and well-being.
"Lost Connections" by Johann Hari: Investigating the causes of depression and anxiety.

Local Support Groups

Check with local mental health organizations or hospitals for in-person or virtual support groups.

Professional Help

Remember, seeking professional help is not only okay, it is important. A licensed therapist, counselor, or psychiatrist can provide personalized guidance and treatment options tailored to your needs.

Acknowledgements

Wow, we've made it to the end of the book. If you are still reading this far, I would first like to thank you. Thank you for taking the time to read my story and braving your storm.

I did not set out to write a book when this project was started. I was at a time in my life when my anxiety had reached an all-time high, and I dug through my toolkit for anything I could use and decided on something I had been told to try but never had - writing. What began as a way to journal my feelings blossomed into an entire book.

That said, there were many times I doubted myself and nearly gave up, so- I would first like to thank each person who continually encouraged me to continue. To those people, who I love more than they can believe- thank you.

Thank you to everyone who read my manuscript as I sculpted and crafted it into a finished piece.

Thank you to everyone who believed in me enough to complete this project, and especially those confident enough to pre-order an advanced copy - your advanced support carried me through the grueling final steps.

To my trio of best friends - you know who you are - thank you for loving and supporting me through not only this journey, but through every hardship I have faced that you have happily carried me through.

And to the people who love me more than the world, thank you for being there for me, always and forever.